# IN THE SHADOWS:
# How to Help Your Seriously Ill Adult Child

by
Patricia Ringos Beach, MSN, RN, AOCN®, ACHPN
and Beth E. White, MSN, RN

Hygeia Media
Pittsburgh, Pennsylvania

ONS Publications Department
Executive Director, Professional Practice and Programs:
Elizabeth M. Wertz Evans, RN, MPM, CPHQ, CPHIMS, FACMPE
Publisher and Director of Publications: Barbara Sigler, RN, MNEd
Managing Editor: Lisa M. George, BA
Technical Content Editor: Angela D. Klimaszewski, RN, MSN
Staff Editor II: Amy Nicoletti, BA
Copy Editor: Laura Pinchot, BA
Graphic Designer: Dany Sjoen

Library of Congress Cataloging-in-Publication Data

Beach, Patricia Ringos.
  In the shadows : how to help your seriously ill adult child / by Patricia Ringos Beach, MSN, RN, AOCN, ACHPN, and Beth E. White, MSN, RN.
    pages cm
  Includes bibliographical references.
  ISBN 978-1-935864-27-1 (alk. paper)
  1. Chronically ill--Family relationships. 2. Caregivers. 3. Adult children--Family relationships. I. White, Beth E. II. Title.
  RC108.B43 2013
  362.16--dc23

                                                          2012041538

### Publisher's Note

This book is published by the Oncology Nursing Society (ONS). ONS neither represents nor guarantees that the practices described herein will, if followed, ensure safe and effective patient care. The recommendations contained in this book reflect ONS's judgment regarding the state of general knowledge and practice in the field as of the date of publication. The recommendations may not be appropriate for use in all circumstances. Those who use this book should make their own determinations regarding specific safe and appropriate patient-care practices, taking into account the personnel, equipment, and practices available at the hospital or other facility at which they are located. The authors and publisher cannot be held responsible for any liability incurred as a consequence from the use or application of any of the contents of this book. Figures and tables are used as examples only. They are not meant to be all-inclusive, nor do they represent endorsement of any particular institution by ONS. Mention of specific products and opinions related to those products do not indicate or imply endorsement by ONS. Web sites mentioned are provided for information only; the hosts are responsible for their own content and availability. Unless otherwise indicated, dollar amounts reflect U.S. dollars.

ONS publications are originally published in English. Publishers wishing to translate ONS publications must contact ONS about licensing arrangements. ONS publications cannot be translated without obtaining written permission from ONS. (Individual tables and figures that are reprinted or adapted require additional permission from the original source.) Because translations from English may not always be accurate or precise, ONS disclaims any responsibility for inaccuracies in words or meaning that may occur as a result of the translation. Readers relying on precise information should check the original English version.

Printed in the United States of America

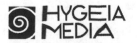

An imprint of the Oncology Nursing Society

To my parents, Rose and Paul Ringos
My daughters, Stacie and Kimberly
My husband, Dan
—*Patricia Ringos Beach*


To Emily and Colleen,
Who have made it possible for me to understand the deep love of a parent for a child.
And
To David, who always believed in me and "the book."
—*Beth E. White*

# Contents

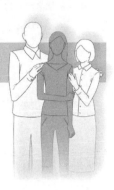

# Acknowledgments

*Write the book you have always wanted to read.*

—Yiyun Li

M any people influenced the writing in this book. It started with the countless patients and their families who we have been privileged to care for as their nurses over the years. They taught us that illness affects not only our patients, but their families. Parents of our patients, both pediatric and adult, openly showed us what we intuitively knew: parental love and devotion do not have an expiration date of 18 or 21 years.

We also acknowledge our colleagues who mentored us and shared in the work we did. They taught us how to practice the art and science of nursing by staying always open to new ideas and appreciating the experiences of those who trusted us with their health. We thank them for encouraging our curiosity.

Because of this support, it just seemed natural to ask anyone who would talk to us about their experiences of parenting beyond childhood.

Over the two years that we researched, interviewed, and wrote this book, there are those who come particularly to mind. These people specifically assisted us to learn about parenting adult children and the most loving and effective ways parents can help when their adult children become seriously ill. In more or less chronological order by their appearance and participation as this book evolved, more than words can say, we are grateful for the help and insights from Joseph Cardone, Myles Sheehan, Barbara Martig, Georgianna Doyle, Amanda Sager, Victoria Raveis, T.J. Symons, Anne Grinyer, Kira Birditt, Karen Fingerman, Aleona Pollauf, Cassie Zak, Renee Charchol and Kathy Schulz, Sandra Cesario, Mohammad Alnsour, Robert Sawicki, George Bonanno, Adelaide Stewart, Sue Deckelman, Charla Ulrich, Lynn Baker, Jamie Kabot with the 4th Angel Patient and Caregiver Mentoring Program, Paulette Rex, Buzz Hermann, Kerrie Berlincourt, Karen Crotte and Eileen Korhumel, Kathy Capps, Sandy Belliveau, Charlotte Scott, Karyn Buxman, Lori Miller and Doreen Joelson, Maxine Young, Lee Williams, Jeanne Kozelek, Nolan Baker, Eric Millhorn, and Mark Clair.

Thank you to our two special readers Maria Nowicki and Cassie Zak. Our heartfelt appreciation goes to Camilla Stanfa who transcribed many hours of interviews.

To all the staff at Hygeia and the Oncology Nursing Society for offering us an opportunity to write a publishable book on a subject that no one talked about by two writers no one had heard of, thank you. May all of us working together produce a product that reaches out to help parents of seriously ill adult children and of which we can be proud.

And, thank you to our families. Thank you for the times other things were put aside or delayed for "the book." The space and support you gave us to work is more valuable than gold. We love you.

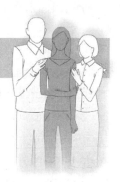

# INTRODUCTION:
# Unexplored
# Territory

*I have found the best way to give advice to your children is to find out what they want and then advise them to do it.*

—Harry Truman

## Debbie's Story

Megan's mom was always there—in the waiting room during clinic appointments and at Megan's bedside when she was hospitalized for problems related to the multiple sclerosis that was diagnosed 18 months ago. We could always depend on Megan's mom. She told the nurses and doctors things that helped them plan care for Megan, like that ever since Megan was a little girl, her stomach felt better when she had ginger ale—at room temperature, and only in a glass, never the can. Megan's mom was so dependable. She picked up Megan's prescriptions and her kids from soccer practice. She dropped off the dry cleaning and cookies for the clinic staff. She made supper for Megan's family so

1

that Megan and her husband could spend time together after work.

It was quite a while before the doctors and nurses learned Megan's mom's name. It was Debbie. Debbie and her second husband moved from an active retirement community in Arizona back to the winters of the Midwest to care for their daughter. Debbie was not really thought of as a mom who needed to be part of her child's care because Megan was an adult.

One day, the doctor asked to speak to Megan and her husband about medical decisions, so Debbie left the room. "Well, I guess they don't need me in there," she said. "They have things to talk about." Her eyes were shiny and her posture a little less erect as she walked to the cafeteria for coffee while the doctor talked to her daughter and son-in-law about important things.

Debbie is an attentive, loving mother who had raised her daughter and launched her into independence more than 10 years ago. Now, this adult child is unexpectedly seriously ill, and an essential support person is left out. Because the doctors and nurses didn't know to offer information, practical aid, or a listening ear to Debbie, she was left in the shadows.

## An Important Social Change

Every generation or so, social changes that seem completely unrelated interact together and result in an entirely new way of looking at how we relate to one another. Sociologists call this radical change *role realignment*; in corporate circles it is called a *paradigm shift*; and Hollywood calls it *the perfect storm*. This kind of paradigm-shifting perfect storm is occurring in health care and family life and is realigning the way we think about parents and grown children. This social change has three parts:

- Older adults are living longer.
- The incidence of serious chronic disease in middle-aged adults is increasing.
- Parents are continuing active involvement in their children's lives well beyond adolescence.

In this second decade of the 21st century, adults are living so much longer that insurance companies are revising actuarial tables. Nearly 50% of adults older than 60 years old have at least one living parent.

At the same time, the huge baby boomer population is being diagnosed with chronic diseases in record numbers. The Centers for Disease Control and Prevention estimate that one-third of middle-aged adults are living with chronic diseases, such as cardiovascular disease, diabetes, chronic lung diseases, and cancer. These are adults who had been healthy as children.

The oldest in society may be the healthier parents of seriously ill, middle-aged adults. It is probably fair to say that when we think about parents of adult children, the general expectation is that as the parent ages and becomes more infirm, the child will become the caregiver for the parent. When the adult child is ill, however, fewer rules of behavior are available to guide the parent. The place in the family for parents in the care of their now grown, independent, but very ill, child is not clear.

Even in health care, this family change was not noticed right away, and there was no sudden realization that the phenomenon was happening. It is hard to say exactly when healthcare professionals began to notice that with increasing frequency, seriously ill adult patients had living parents. These parents were relatively healthy and seemed to help our patients and their families in many ways. They were present in the hospital and during outpatient treatments. Usually, they were quiet. When they asked questions, it was typically in a respectful and slightly hesitant way. When planning care for adult patients, healthcare providers usually label parents as "support systems" or "family resources" because parents helped the patients by shopping and caring for grandchildren and driving to clinic appointments. They were quiet helpers, not decision makers. They were in the shadows.

Over time, it became obvious. These important family members were not getting the help they needed. Surely adult children expected different things from their parents than minor children, but those expectations were not well known. Understanding of parental desire to assist their adult children was nearly absent. Some of these answers depended on the age and independence level of the child and the closeness of the relationship. Certainly, common sense and intuition implied that the parent-child bond remained strong even when the child was grown.

Not much is known about how parents could best relate to children as mature adults rather than as dependent immature children. Books and Web sites that address parent and adult child relationships largely send conflicting messages: *Let adult children plan their own lives. If you help them too much, they will resent you. Stand by, however, because your adult children often call upon you for assistance. Be friendly, but not their friend.* Adult children and parents were left to follow unspecified guidelines.

Even less is known about the experience of navigating the healthcare system with an adult child who had established independence from parents and was now very sick. What was known led to more questions than answers. How were parents supposed to behave with their child's spouse? Given strict laws governing the privacy of health information, how much and what kind of information should parents expect? How much help was enough? What kind of help was needed and most appreciated? Did parent age matter? Did the child's age matter?

A few parents were forthcoming. Casual comments ranged from resigned to resentful to guilty to gratitude for the ability to help: "I thought this was *my* time. I didn't expect to come out of retirement to take care of my kids again." "What can you do? He's my son, after all." "Do you think I caused the breast cancer? It does run in my side of the family." "Thank goodness I am healthy enough to help out. I would do anything for her and her family."

## Historical Perspective on Parenting

Because professional experts were few, it became obvious that the real experts needed to be consulted: the parents of seriously ill adult children. But first, a historical perspective on parenting and health care was needed. The past three generations of parents, more than generations before them, anticipate continued close involvement with adult children. Understanding what influenced those parents when their children were young was essential to understanding why continued attachment was valued, even expected. Interest in parenting started in earnest right after World War II.

Drs. Benjamin Spock and Jonas Salk greatly influenced the parenting movement. Dr. Spock was the first popular expert on what we have come to call good parenting. Dr. Salk's research successes provided evidence that we could believe in the near infallibility of modern medicine to keep children alive and healthy to adulthood.

Dr. Spock, the pediatrician who came on the national scene right after World War II, delivered a most controversial message: Children are not just little adults. They are unique individuals.

In his book *Baby and Child Care* (1946), Dr. Spock told parents that just feeding, clothing, and telling children to follow the rules was not good enough. Children need love. Don't worry about spoiling your children. Raising children was an important job, maybe the most important job ever, Dr. Spock told parents.

America was ready to listen. World War II was over and the economy was on the upswing. Prosperity, along with respect for the job needs of returning veterans, made it possible for moms to stay home and care for the kids while dads worked. There was a boom in births. Raising baby boomer children took on importance because it was one outcome that stay-at-home moms could point to as evidence of their worth.

Dr. Spock poured a solid foundation, but he was just the beginning. Children and parents began to be studied in earnest. Baby boomer children were arguably the first generation who were openly loved and cherished—and studied—by society. Names such as Thomas Gordon (2011a, 2011b), Don Dinkmeyer Sr., Gary McKay, and Don Dinkmeyer Jr. (2007), and James Dobson (1997–2012) became widely recognized. These psychologists, clergy, and social scientists gave parents skills to effectively communicate with and discipline children. They each carried a similar message: Being a parent takes new knowledge. Being a parent requires skills and purposeful action. You are not just born with the ability to be a good parent. You have to be purposeful about it. You need to understand growth and development. Children need to be pruned, not yanked, supported and encouraged, not punished and ridiculed

In fact, being a parent required a new word: "Parenting" became an active verb. Parenting has come to mean thoughtfully considering family values and the developmental stage of each child to foster self-esteem, intellectual curiosity, and regard for others. Because parenting is a job, parents must need skills. Parents began taking parenting classes with acronyms such as PET (Parent Effectiveness Training) (Gordon, 2011a), FET (Family Effectiveness Training) (Gordon, 2011b), and STEP (Systematic Training for Effective Parenting) (Dinkmeyer et al., 2007). The trend continues. Women's magazines almost always have at least one article on effective parenting. Churches and community centers offer classes on parent-child communication, disciplining with love, natural and logical consequences, Mommy and Me, parenting teenagers, parenting by the Bible, and so much more. Ever since Dr. Spock gave parents of baby boomers the charge to raise children well, parents have been asking: How can I tell if I'm a good parent? What should I do to nurture my child? What is good-enough discipline? Is spanking OK? Would my child be OK if I bottle fed him? Would my child be ruined if I went back to work? Should I communicate with my child as though I am in charge or as though our home is a democracy, or is befriending my child

the best approach? Intense discussions about parent-child relationships occur in popular magazines and professional journals, at parent-teacher organization meetings and backyard
barbecues. Parenting Web sites and blogs were created to give
parents a forum to discuss ideas and worries about raising
young children.

Over the past 65 years, the message has only become clearer
and more refined: a young child becomes a successful adult by
developing self-confidence and positive social relationships.
The foundation of all child development rests on genetics and
the first relationship of all, the child and the parent. Guilt has
become a part of every parent's life.

Parents race toward the prize: graduation and independence, and hopefully, a good job and marriage, and pray God,
healthy grandchildren. The children were raised. The job is
done.

And then, the advice . . . almost . . . completely . . . stops.

Parents of adult children don't have many guideposts on
the journey to a "grown-up" relationship with their independent children. The most consistent advice for parents is a bit
like this: Don't give advice, and don't appear too needy and
hope the kids keep coming around. This kind of parenting
advice does not give much guidance when grown children become very ill and dependent.

Parents invest a great deal of themselves into raising children. Even when children have been independent for many
years, the bond continues. In the words of Toni Morrison
(2006), "Grown don't mean nothing to a mother. A child is a
child. They get bigger, older, but grown? What's that supposed
to mean? In my heart, it don't mean a thing" (p. 57).

## Medical Miracles and Parenting

Parents have the luxury to focus on the emotional side of parenting because of medical pioneers like Dr. Salk. Jonas Salk, MD, was a physician and medical researcher who developed the polio vaccine. Although the polio vaccine was not the first vaccine, it was developed in the 1950s when summertime was a time of anxiety and fear for parents of baby boomers. Polio, or *poliomyelitis*, is a crippling and life-threatening disease that infected children most often in the summer. This highly contagious disease attacks the central nervous system and is spread by eating or drinking the polio virus. Epidemics typically occur in warmer climates and when groups of people are active. The combination of spirited outdoor activity with friends coupled with summer temperatures made children susceptible to infection (Nichols, 2012). Polio affected many thousands of children every year. Whole communities isolated children in the summer. Parents felt powerless and frightened. The polio vaccine lifted that fear. Medical science came through (Kluger, 2004).

Dr. Salk was certainly not the only medical scientist working on amazing treatments to control and prevent disease. He is only one of the most famous because most baby boomers remember standing in long lines at schools or churches to get a shot or a sugar cube to prevent a paralyzing disease.

Amazing medical breakthroughs have occurred since the second half of the 20th century. Babies who would have died even a generation ago are alive and well today because of advances in newborn care. Today, some cancers are curable, and most are treatable and result in chronic illness rather than an automatic death sentence. Diabetes is controllable. Drugs that keep cholesterol levels low, blood pressure down, and damaged lungs functioning are commonplace. Medical science can hold at bay the results of our poor lifestyles. DNA was discovered in the 1950s. Genes were mapped, and then amazingly the exact locations of some disease-producing chromosomes were found on genes. Some diseases can be diagnosed before birth and treated immediately after birth. Some conditions can even be treated before birth with prenatal surgery.

Whether ill or healthy, people have been encouraged to learn about their health. The popular phrase is "advocate for yourself." Ask questions. Expect to participate in decisions with your healthcare provider. Check the Internet. Ask your healthcare providers for written information about everything prescribed or diagnosed. Get a second opinion. Read your chart. *You* are in charge of *your* health.

With all that medical success and all those self-affirming mantras, it is understandable that we may have the illusion that all diseases can be cured, or at least treated for a very long time. If a disease does not respond, the problem must be the doctor's fault or the person is not fighting the disease hard enough. In the words of Fr. Joseph Cardone, a Roman Catholic priest (personal communication, June 16, 2010), "some of us even think medicine has made death optional."

Drs. Spock and Salk have taught us two important lessons. First, willingly or reluctantly, once a parent, always a parent. Second, parents of children of every age look to the healthcare system to help make things better. Parents of young children expect to be included in medical decision making when their children are ill. Parents of adult children want to be included, but don't know what to do or how to behave.

# Debbie's Story

Debbie's need to parent her seriously ill adult child was not well understood by her daughter or the healthcare team. When she asked Megan and her husband if she could listen in when they talked to the doctors, she was pleased with their response. Although her role continues to be supportive, Debbie now feels as though she is an important part of her daughter's medical treatment plan.

# Conclusion

*In the Shadows. How to Help Your Seriously Ill Adult Child* is a book of stories, evidence, and advice that is the result of hours of interviews with parents, their ill adult children, and professionals. The parents' stories are accounts of real people told as faithfully as possible but with identifying details and names changed. When asked, parents were eager to talk and tell their story. They would explain what their experience was like and what they wish healthcare providers could have done to help them. They gave advice for friends and other family members. Some lessons were hard to learn. These parents asked that their stories be shared in the hope that their perspectives will help others find some guidance to support their ill adult child and themselves.

The insights and resources are described in 10 chapters. Chapter topics include parenting adult children, your other important relationships, emotional responses to having an ill child, providing physical care to your ill child, financial concerns in serious illness, caring for yourself, communication challenges when serious illness occurs, how spirituality may help you cope, navigating the healthcare system, and coping with your child's prognosis.

Having an ill child of any age is difficult. May these stories and advice shed light for you and your family. You are not alone in this journey. We wish to help you move from the shadows as you and your child live your own story.

# References

Dinkmeyer, D., Sr., McKay, G.D., & Dinkmeyer, D., Jr. (2007). *The parent's handbook: Systematic training for effective parenting.* Fredericksburg, VA: STEP Publishers.

Dobson, J. (1997–2012). Focus on the Family parenting ministry. Retrieved from    http://www.focusonthefamily.com/parenting/articles/parenting _ministry.aspx

Gordon, T. (2011a). Family effectiveness training (F.E.T.). Retrieved from http://www.gordontraining.com/parent-programs/family-effectiveness -training-f-e-t

Gordon, T. (2011b). Parent effectiveness training (P.E.T.). Retrieved from http://www.gordontraining.com/parent-programs/parent-effectiveness -training-p-e-t

Kluger, J. (2004). *The splendid solution: Jonas Salk and the conquest of polio.* New York, NY: Penguin.

Morrison, T. (2006). *Beloved.* New York, NY: Alfred A. Knopf.

Nichols, J.F. (2012, January). Polio: Perspective of a polio survivor. Re- trieved from    http://www.chop.edu/service/parents-possessing-accessing -communicating-knowledge-about-vaccines/vaccine-preventable-diseases/ polio.html

Spock, B. (1946). *The common sense book of baby and child care.* New York, NY: Duell, Sloan and Pearce.

# CHAPTER 1

# ONCE A PARENT, ALWAYS A PARENT:
# Exploring the Parent-Child Relationship

*We've had bad luck with children; they've all grown up.*
—Christopher Morley

## Lisa's Story

I t's the second Tuesday of the month. Heather, a 45-year-old married woman and mother of three teenagers, is in the outpatient clinic to receive one of the medications that everyone fervently hopes will shrink her ovarian tumors and prolong her life. Heather hates the medication that is given in a special IV port in her shoulder. It makes her feel nauseated, moody, and utterly exhausted. No one knows if Heather is going to be pleasant today or angry at the world. The chemotherapy nurses and the oncology team of social workers and clergy are trained to care for these emotional ups and downs, but they only need to contend with her for a few hours each month.

Sitting next to Heather in the treatment bay is a 66-year-old woman wearing a stylish sweater set, jeans, and leather boots. This is Heather's mother, Lisa. Lisa drives Heather to these clinic appointments because Heather can't drive afterward and her son-in-law has to work. Lisa listens as Heather complains about her circumstances. She makes the grocery list while Heather naps during treatment. Besides, she asks, "Who else should be doing this?"

Lisa is recently retired; she was a bank manager for more than two decades. She is not shy about asserting herself. Every second Tuesday of the month, Lisa waits for Heather's doctor. When the young oncology physician comes in to examine Heather, it is obvious that he is trying to avoid Lisa's gaze. He leaves the room and quickly seeks the refuge of the nurses' station, but Lisa catches him in the hallway. "How is she doing, Doctor?" "What do you think her chances are? Is she any better than last month?"

The doctor explains today, as he has done every month, that he is not permitted to give private information to Lisa without Heather's knowledge. He reminds Lisa of the federal privacy laws, as well as his respect for Heather as an adult patient who makes her own decisions.

Lisa's voice rises slightly as she says, "But she is sick, and I am her mother. I should have a right to know about my daughter's health. You are treating me like I'm some bystander. I am still her mother!"

## Parenting: The Feelings Never Stop

"I am still her mother!" Lisa's plea begs for understanding that parental feelings don't evaporate when children grow up.

Lisa's frustrations are shared by many parents of seriously ill adult children.

"I didn't know what I was supposed to act like," said Ally, whose 42-year-old son has traumatic brain injury following a motor vehicle crash. "But, I love my child and want to be part of his life."

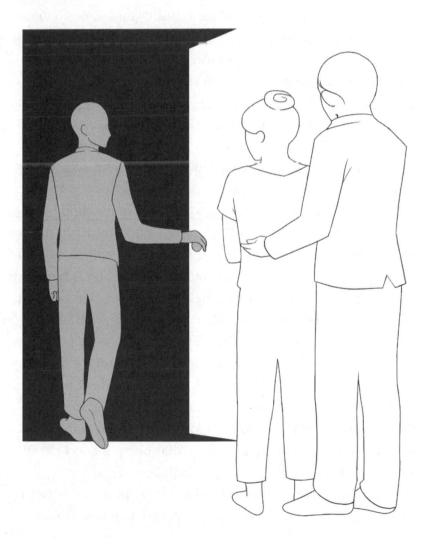

Brenda, the parent of a 54-year-old woman who has suffered a series of strokes, said, "I'm so grateful when my daughter and her husband let me in to talk with the doctors and help make decisions. I know they trust my judgment. But, I have to tread lightly. I don't want them to resent me or think I'm interfering."

"I was treated all over the place," said Diane, whose daughter developed ovarian cancer when a second-year law student. "Sometimes, the nurses were kind and included me in their care, and sometimes I heard the doctors and nurses refer to me as The Mother."

Lisa, Ally, Brenda, and Diane know that "once a parent, always a parent." But they, similar to many parents, didn't know exactly what it means to be a parent when children are adults— and especially when children are adults and seriously ill.

Parents don't know how to act when their adult child is very ill. They report that they are often relegated from the most important person in a child's life to someone who is treated like extended family. Parents certainly figured it out when the children were younger. Heaven help the pediatrician that did not call a worried parent quickly enough! It can't be that parents give up involvement in their children's lives when a child is grown. Parents of young to middle-aged adults expect to continue to be part of their children's lives beyond the time that children reach the age of maturity. These mothers and fathers became parents in the Dr. Spock era. Dr. Benjamin Spock helped mothers and fathers believe that being a good parent was a measurement of being a good adult.

The topic of parenting has staying power probably because parenting affects everyone. Everyone had parents. For most people, the first loving relationship was with a parenting adult, whether biologic, adoptive, or foster. This relationship is so emotionally binding and life-lasting that it is nearly impossible to describe it. For better or for worse, the parent–young child relationship affects the way people of all ages relate to others.

Parenting takes on an even more profound meaning when people become parents. Identification and attachment to children is probably the deepest relationship most will ever know. Parents want to know what makes a "good parent" and the tricks of the trade that will result in a "good kid." Almost all parents look for ways to make the next generations better. "Our children give us the opportunity to become the parents we always wished we'd had," said psychologist Louise Hart (Kuzma, 1997, p. 31).

It is generally believed that a parent's job is to make children independent. Parents have done their job well when children grow up to be independent, successful, and responsible. This usually translates into "get a job, find a nice mate, and contribute to the well-being of the community . . . and some healthy grandchildren, please."

Does this mean that parents are supposed to focus efforts so that children do not need them so much anymore? Actually, yes. The reasoning is this: a parent's job is to ensure that the children are safely brought to maturity. Once children are "launched" or living independently, parents generally recognize that their importance in their children's lives will diminish. Most expect they will probably remain a helper during times of struggle. After all, many parents have been asked by their adult children to babysit, float a loan for a new car, or listen to tirades about the horrible behavior of their child's boss.

Most parents would report they were happy to do it. But essentially, adult children are supposed to make their own lives. Then, the parenting job is finished until old age. Eventually, the tables will turn and adult children will become the caregivers for parents when frailty begins.

Most of what is known about parenting comes from research at both ends of the parenting spectrum: raising children to adulthood on the left, and being cared for by children in old age on the right. By far, the largest volume of parenting research is about the challenges of raising children from birth to age 18 or so. At the other end of the parent-child spectrum, a fair amount of study and conversation occurs about children caring for elderly parents. Adult child caregivers can access information about legal powers of attorney, daycare resources for their parents, and community and online discussions with others caring for elderly parents.

Little guidance is offered to parents in the middle of the parenting spectrum—decades between when children take on adult roles and the time when parents become infirm. This is the time when parents are still working or actively retired, and adult children are establishing their independent lives. The proper role of the parent-child relationship during these years is less clear. Typical expectations for parent–adult child attachment are not well understood. Some parents expect to be closely involved in children's adult lives, whereas others believe that is too invasive. Some parents wish to become friends with their adult children, and others do not believe that is even possible. Parents may expect to have a say in the big decisions of children's adult lives. Other parents think it best to wait to be asked. When parents have retired and are now traveling or otherwise enjoying the fruits of the working years, they may wonder if it is appropriate to expect that their lives may be interrupted to care for an ill adult child.

These concerns have not been talked about very much. No wonder that parents don't know how to help adult children who are really sick.

Just as parents look for expert advice when children are young, so can parents of adult children benefit from four Adult Child Parenting Guidelines when children are older.

## Adult Child Parenting Guideline #1: Growth and Development Is Not Just for Little Kids

Growth and development continues throughout life. A short review of growth and development beyond childhood can be reassuring. Everyone struggles through the various life stages. Probably no one has explained the tug and pull of each stage as simply and clearly as Erik Erikson (Harder, 2011). Erikson described emotional growth and development from infancy through old age. Through every stage, everyone has a chance to deepen relationships with others and find life satisfaction. At each stage, different challenges must be overcome and different events are important. Reviewing these stages helps clarify the maturation of human relationships beginning with the trust an infant has with his mother and father and continuing in childhood through development of independence in adolescence and through adult years. The stages of growth and development can also explain why parents' well-meaning approaches to adult children may not be understood or well received.

It is important to remember that life stage affects the way people view one another. Here is where Erikson makes a very important point: life stage will always be different for parents and children. Parents will never be at the same stage of development as their children, no matter the age. When looked at through this lens, it becomes clearer how parents might "fit" into adult children's lives (Wethington & Kamp Dush, 2007).

For example, during the young adult to early middle years of life, adults are typically interested in creating meaningful relationships at work and at home. Activity centers on maintaining a loving relationship with another (non-parent) adult, making a career and home, and perhaps raising children. The focus is looking outward. This point of view is different from adults who are in the late middle-to-older age group when the focus is on looking inward. Retirement begins. Lifetime accomplishments are reviewed, and meaningful time spent in sharing lessons learned with peers and the youngest generation is most important for emotional health.

Understanding the normal developmental viewpoints of differently aged adults brings an appreciation of relationships with adult children. The age appropriateness of adult children's focus on spouses or careers or their own children is better understood when life stage is considered. Taking growth and development into account will help parents begin to understand why a child's spouse, young children, or career needs and desires take priority. For example, running errands may be the best way to help adult children when they are very ill: this task may allow them to continue to work on a project at work or give them the strength to read a story to their children. Just as parents benefited by understanding how to cope with temper tantrums when their children were toddlers, so is the parent role strengthened when developmental needs of adults are considered when their children are grown. However, even the most developmentally astute parents have days when they feel less than fully supportive of their very ill adult child, which is why Adult Child Parenting Guideline #2 is needed.

## Adult Child Parenting Guideline #2: Tension in Parent and Adult Child Relationships Is Normal

A small but influential number of social scientists are studying parent and adult child relationships. They include Kira Birditt of the University of Michigan (Birditt, Fingerman, Lefkowitz, & Kamp Dush, 2008; Birditt, Fingerman, & Zarit, 2010) and Karen Fingerman of Purdue University (Fingerman, 2000, 2001, 2003; Fingerman, Chen, Hay, Cichy, & Lefkowitz, 2006), who characterize the adult child and parent relationship as one in which tension can be expected. Drs. Birditt and Fingerman call this tension *ambivalence*. Ambivalence refers to having high positive and negative feelings about the same relationship. Ambivalence includes feelings of irritation and tension alongside love and affection. "In any close relationship there is a push and pull for independence and closeness. The struggle seems to be especially strong in parent–adult child relationships," said Dr. Birditt (personal communication, August 26, 2010). Adult children must be treated as adults, but the relationship is not the same as with other adults in the parents' lives. Dr. Anne Grinyer of Lancaster University (personal communication, August 20, 2010) also reported this from Great

Britain. Dr. Grinyer found that tension could be very high, especially when adult children are newly independent and feel that parents are demanding and not allowing freedom from parental oversight.

Parents might feel ambivalence differently with different children. If adult children are successful, parents tend to feel proud and close to them. Unsuccessful children can cause sadness, but not always. Parents may also feel closer to children who have problems, especially problems that are not their fault, such as illness (Greenfield & Marks, 2006).

Ambivalence continues throughout adult life. Because parents will always be at a different developmental stage than their child, the preferred ways to share closeness will be different for most of the parent's and child's lives. When in their early-to-mid-20s, children who want their parents to join in the joy of their newly discovered independence are common. This is typically a self-centered time in young adult life, yet it comes at a stage in a parent's life when an outward focus takes priority, such as active involvement in social and community life. Some parents report enjoying their young adult's pleasure by remembering the thrill of life's prospects unfolding, and some may feel a little annoyed because their attentions are elsewhere. Whenever an adult child or a parent is perceived as being too demanding, ambivalence may result.

Ambivalence does not mean parents don't love their adult children and want the best for them. Ambivalence does not mean adult children do not love their parents or have concern about their well-being. Ambivalence comes from differing priorities within a very close and very meaningful relationship (Luscher & Pillemer, 2004).

What may be true is that ambivalence is perceived as more troublesome for parents than it is for children. This leads to discussion of the sometimes controversial Adult Child Parenting Guideline #3.

## Adult Child Parenting Guideline #3: The Love Between Parents and Children Is Not Equal

This guideline is shocking to some. Indeed, it is very seldom spoken out loud. Perhaps parents have trouble experiencing conflicting, ambivalent feelings toward their children because parents love their children more than children love their parents.

This does not mean that adult children do not love parents, nor does it mean that adult children do not respond to crises and come to their parents' aid. It does mean that although the occasional child will devote his life to the care of an ill parent, our society does not necessarily expect that level of sacrifice and devotion. The expectation is different when an adult child is very ill. As Adeline said, "I know some women who have ill husbands, and they keep on going to bridge club and golf. No one in my support group who has ill adult children has been able to keep up with their previous social commitments."

The parent's bond to the child is strong and forever and not equal. The adult child's bond to the parent may be strong and close, but it is not of the same intensity. The parent's bond to the child is the "lying down in front of the bus" kind of love. This may explain why parents have stronger feelings in every respect when children are very ill. Feelings are strong and range from the very positive to negative. Parents report feeling more irritation but more closeness, and more anger but more forgiveness. This is completely normal. Adult Child Parenting Guideline #4 discusses how to find support for those feelings.

## Adult Child Parenting Guideline #4: When Adult Children Are Seriously Ill, All Parents Need a Support System

Just because these negative feelings are normal does not mean they are for the good or that they should be expressed unchecked or hidden away. Because these feelings are so wide and intense, it is a good idea to learn how to cope with am- bivalence and irritation. Relationship tensions are associated with the underlying quality of the parent-child relationship. In addition, parents and adult children often describe differ- ing perceptions of ambivalence and conflict with parents. De- velopmental stage influences the degree of reported ambiva- lence. During transition periods, such as adolescence to young adult, ambivalence tends to be high. Some researchers have found that parents always have more emotional investment in adult children, whereas others have found that the age and stage of the parent and child better predicts the degree of con- flict (Birditt & Fingerman, 2011; Birditt, Miller, Fingerman, & Lefkowitz, 2009; Buhl, 2008). In any case, when conflict occurs, if there is a lot of yelling and screaming, or conversely, a lot of stony silence, the relationship quality becomes poor, and par- ents can actually become sick. Resolution has the best chance if parents open the door by admitting an issue exists, find a way to talk it through, and listen to their adult child and other important people in his life, such as his spouse. Parents are often the leaders to try to find a solution that works for everybody.

This sounds a lot easier than it often is. One of the benefits of being able to look back over the total experience of raising children is that it is easier to convince parents that support from other parents may be just as important now as it was when the children were younger. Most parents *of every age* find that contact with other parents who are going through a similar situation is invaluable.

The support groups used when children were young were found in places like parent-teacher organizations, the daycare center, and the children's church program. When children are grown, finding access to people in a comparable situation is not simple. When a friend or a group is found who will listen and help, parents should embrace them (literally!) and be thankful. But, what if this kind of support is not available? Increasingly, parents are saying that they are turning to technology, specifically the Internet, for support.

Adults of all ages are becoming more technologically savvy. Knowledge can be shared and problems aired as easily across the country as across the back fence. E-mail, smartphones, and texting are commonplace. *Blogs* (short for Web log), online diaries or opinion pages, are common and widely shared. Skype and FaceTime allow users to see and talk to distant friends and family in real time. Searching for information on the Internet is as common as looking in a dictionary or an encyclopedia was a generation ago. Although it is relatively easy to type in a word or phrase and have a search engine suggest a few million "hits," it takes some sophistication to know how to evaluate the information on those many Web sites. It is important to have some way to discern what is truth and what is hooey and to be able to evaluate whether the information is a come-on to get you to buy something or is freely offered and useful.

Online parent support groups are increasing in number and can be found through conversations with healthcare providers, clergy, and social workers and by simply typing in a desired group in your browser and clicking "Search." Searches may be conducted about diseases, such as "support groups multiple sclerosis" or "ill adult children blog" or similar terms and combinations. Because anyone who has a computer and an opinion can open up an online support group or Web site, it is essential that you know how to evaluate these sites. Specific suggestions are found in the "By the Way…" section at the end of this chapter.

Online support groups are anonymous, which some parents find reassuring. Being able to share your issues without worry about judgment is often cathartic. Elizabeth Edwards (2009), in her book *Resilience*, talked about the relief she felt when talking to anonymous online parents who understood the pain of losing a child but did not hold her to any different standard because they didn't know she was the wife of a U.S. senator and presidential candidate. They only knew her as Elizabeth who lost a son.

Some cautions about Internet support groups are in order. Not all sites will practice the same values or perspectives. If a site is offensive, simply stop going to that site. Be very cautious about disclosing personal information such as your address or phone numbers or other identifying information that could allow others to track your location. Don't send money. Otherwise, use this technology to your advantage.

## Lisa's Story

Lisa needed support and recognized that her very ill daughter was too emotionally fragile to be that resource. Lisa also knew she needed to talk to other parents who had a life stage perspective similar to hers. Lisa applied the organizational and analytical skills that served her well in the business world. She found a face-to-face support group in her community that meets twice a month in a local coffee shop. She also participates in an online ovarian cancer chat room where she can learn about progress in the treatment of this disease and get emotional support any time of the day or night.

## Conclusion

Parents and adult children will have different relationships with one another depending on the life stage of each. Ambivalent feelings toward adult children often catch parents by surprise, especially if the child is ill "through no fault of their own." It is normal for parents to feel stronger love toward their children *at every age.* A serious illness affects both the adult child and the parent. Understanding the growth and development of adults and the unique nature of adult child–parent relationships can help families to anticipate potential conflicts so they can be resolved promptly or avoided. It is possible to learn about parent relationships with adult children in sickness and in health by talking to each other. When you feel understood and supported, you can focus your attention on a united family-centered approach to treating the serious illness rather than family alienation.

# References

Birditt, K.S., & Fingerman, K.L. (2011). Relationships between adults and aging parents. In K. Warner Schaie & S.L. Willis (Eds.), *Handbook of the psychology of aging* (7th ed., pp. 219–228). New York, NY: Elsevier.

Birditt, K.S., Fingerman, K.L., Lefkowitz, E.S., & Kamp Dush, C.M. (2008). Parents perceived as peers: Filial maturity in adulthood. *Journal of Adult Development, 15*, 1–12. doi:10.1007/s10804-007-9019-2

Birditt, K.S., Fingerman, K.L., & Zarit, S.H. (2010). Adult children's problems and successes: Implications for intergenerational ambivalence. *Journals of Gerontology: Series B Psychological Sciences and Social Sciences, 65B*, 145–153. doi:10.1093/geronb/gbp125

Birditt, K.S., Miller, L.M., Fingerman, K.L., & Lefkowitz, E.S. (2009). Tension in the parent and adult child relationship: Links to solidarity and ambivalence. *Psychology and Aging, 24*, 289–295. doi:10.1037/a0015196

Buhl, H.M. (2008). Significance of individuation in adult child-parent relationships. *Journal of Family Issues, 29*, 262–281. doi:10.1177/0192513X07304272

Edwards, E. (2009). *Resilience: Reflections on the burdens and gifts of facing life's adversities.* New York, NY: Crown Publishing Group.

Fingerman, K.L. (2000). "We had a nice little chat": Age and generational differences in mothers' and daughters' descriptions of enjoyable visits. *Journals of Gerontology: Series B Psychological Sciences and Social Sciences, 55B*, 95–106. doi:10.1093/geronb/55.2.P95

Fingerman, K.L. (2001). A distant closeness: Intimacy between parents and their children in later life. *Generations, 25*(2), 26–33.

Fingerman, K.L. (2003). *Mothers and their adult daughters: Mixed emotions, enduring bonds.* Amherst, NY: Prometheus.

Fingerman, K.L., Chen, P.C., Hay, E., Cichy, K.E., & Lefkowitz, E.S. (2006). Ambivalent reactions in the parent and offspring relationship. *Journals of Gerontology: Series B Psychological Sciences and Social Sciences, 61B*, 152–160. doi:10.1093/geronb/61.3.P152

Greenfield, E.A., & Marks, N.F. (2006). Linked lives: Adult children's problems and their parents' psychological and relational well-being. *Journal of Marriage and Family, 68*, 442–454. doi:10.1111/j.1741-3737.2006.00263.x

Harder, A.F. (2011, August 11). The developmental stages of Erik Erikson. Retrieved from http://www.support4change.com/index.php?option=com_k2&view=item&id=47;erik-erikson-developmental-stages

Kuzma, K. (1997). *Easy obedience: Teaching children self-discipline with love.* Hagerstown, MD: Review and Herald Publishing Association.

Luscher, K., & Pillemer, K. (2004). *Intergenerational ambivalences: New perspectives on parent-child relations in later life.* Ithaca, NY: Elsevier.

Wethington, E., & Kamp Dush, C.M. (2007). Assessments of parenting quality and experiences across the life course. *Advances in Life Course Research, 12,* 123–152. doi:10.1016/S1040-2608(07)12005-0

**By the Way...**

**Using the Internet: Finding It Is Only Half the Battle
Learning to Evaluate Web-Based Resources**

The Web is one of the best ways to learn from each other about how to be the best parents when children are grown. It is important when children are healthy. It may be a lifeline when adult children are seriously ill.

The basics of evaluating a Web site are very similar to those you would use if you were evaluating a library book, magazine article, or newspaper resource. If you are watching a video on the Internet, you can also look at facial expressions and the setting for the video to give you hints. Here is a list of some of the ways you can evaluate resources on the Web.

- Can you tell who sponsored the site? Is this a for-profit or not-for-profit site? Is the sponsor a well-known and respected one?
- Did the site come up on your screen under the heading *Sponsored Site*? Sponsored Sites pay money to be on the search engine and may be looking to sell a product or service in exchange for some information.
- Is the information credible based on your knowledge and experience?
- If you are not familiar with the information, can you find whom to contact for more information?
- Is the author an expert? What are his or her credentials?
- Does the site have links (highlighted areas you can click on to find more information)? Are the links pertinent?
- When was the site last updated?
- Does the site ask you for personal information before you are allowed access to it? You may or may not feel safe providing information that is easy to obtain, such as your e-mail address. Caution is urged for sites that ask for personal identifying information and credit card or Social Security numbers. This rule is the same as it would be for any other face-to-face transaction you might have. Think about it: if a man showed up at your front door selling something, you would not give him your credit card number, or if a woman at the mall told you she had the secret to happiness, you wouldn't give her your Social Security number and home address, would you?
- What is the point of view of the site? Is it consistent with your values and beliefs?

Web sites are not permanent fixtures on the Internet. They may be available one week and gone the next. Just as businesses at your local mall may be open this month and closed the next time you visit, so do Web sites open and close. With that caution, here are a few Web sites about parenting that you may find interesting and helpful:

- Parenting Grown Children: What Dr. Spock Forgot to Tell Us: www.grownchildren.net
- Helium. How to Relate to Adult Children: www.helium.com/knowledge/580842-how-to-relate-to-adult-children
- Empowering Parents. Parenting Articles About Adult Children: www.empoweringparents.com/category-adult-children.php
- Focus on the Family. Parenting Adult Children: www.focusonthefamily.com/parenting/parenting_roles/parenting-adult-children.aspx
- Ill Adult Children: www.illadultchildren.com

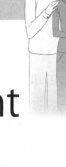

# CHAPTER 2

# YOU ARE NOT ALONE:
# Other Important Relationships

> *Consider a new beginning with your family—choose to take them less seriously. Love them as they are, and forgive them everything.*
>
> —Jonathan Lockwood Huie

## Loretta's Story

Lori is a 36-year-old married woman who has colon cancer. Her mother, Loretta, lives with her husband 1,500 miles away. Loretta has come to stay at Lori's house to care for Lori's children after Lori's surgeries and during the rough spots of chemotherapy. She comes every few weeks and stays for about five to seven days. Lori is grateful to her mother for helping during this challenging time. When Loretta is there, Lori's household continues to run smoothly and Sean, Lori's husband, can concentrate on his career and supporting his ill wife.

Loretta, though, feels tugged at by many others. Important relationships are pulling her back to her home. Her husband, her other adult children, grandchildren, and even her book club friends are asking when she will be back home to spend time with them. They all want to know how Lori is doing, but Loretta feels that she is saying the same thing over and over to everyone. Truthfully, she is tired. She is no longer accustomed to meeting the needs of a growing family on a day-to-day basis. Her other grown children and husband at home are sounding a bit jealous of the time she is spending with Lori. How can Loretta balance her desire to be present with her ill child and also sustain her other relationships?

## Other Important Relationships

Illness changes families. The new normal is uncertainty. Perhaps you consider yourself a stable, clear-thinking person with strong morals and rock-solid convictions. Perhaps you think of yourself as a flexible individual, able to easily cope with change. Even so, when serious illness affects your deeply loved child, you may find yourself making exceptions. You may find yourself considering decisions that you never thought were acceptable. Decisions are often harder to make. Sometimes choices seem scarce; sometimes the number of choices seems overwhelming. When a trauma such as a serious illness occurs, reactions are not typical. Your reaction can change even within the same situation when illness events occur. When the traumatic situation includes a child of any age, parental reactions threaten to become even more unpredictable. You may not be the self you have come to trust. Your world has been turned upside down. You could use words of encouragement and hope.

Yet, your fears and worries may be overlooked. Because you are the mom or dad, you may be expected to do what you have always done. Know what to do. Understand what is expected without being told. To paraphrase a common expression, it does take a village to take care of a sick family member. You may find that you are appointed the Head Servant of the Village, or you may feel like your assignment is the Ignored One Outside the City Gates. Regardless, your communication with your ill adult child's spouse and children, your other children, your spouse, extended family, and your friends will be carefully scrutinized and evaluated by others.

In this chapter, parents and family experts will tell you about giving and receiving support from the other important people in your life. You'll find some encouraging news about communication skills in midlife and some positive ways to hold families (and yourself) together when your child is very ill, as well as some definite landmines to avoid. The parents learned some tough lessons, but looking back, the right path was more obvious than they had originally thought.

## Balanced Connection

Finding the right balance between too much and too little connection with your ill adult child can be tricky. Michelle Miller-Day (2004) studied the relationships among three generations of adult women: mothers, adult daughters, and grandmothers. She found that a well-functioning family depended on appreciating the developmental stage of the parent and the child. A parent who exerts too much control may be seen in a power struggle with her daughter. A person caught in a power struggle may avoid contact or simply acquiesce. Either reaction diminishes the adult child's independence or autonomy. Miller-Day found a similar response when privacy barriers were breached. Mothers who spoke indiscriminately about life's intimate details found themselves less trusted and more likely to be left out. In other words, openness was valued between generations only if it was perceived that personal business was not arbitrarily shared. Miller-Day (2004) found families worked best if mothers recognized their adult child's need for independence. Furthermore, supporting the child's responsibility for decision making seemed to support the need to depend on family members to value one another's experiences.

The good news about Miller-Day's work is that people who are in the midlife years are better able to effectively communicate than at any other age. Other researchers have found that midlife communication is more patient and less argumentative (Fingerman, Nussbaum, & Birditt, 2004).

## Midlife Communication

Trying to categorize the behavior of a very large group of people is an impossible task. All parents of seriously ill adult children do not behave exactly the same way. Yet researchers have found that the behavior of middle-aged adults showed some important patterns over many studies and many years (Birditt & Fingerman, 2005; Fingerman & Birditt, 2003; Fingerman et al., 2004). Interestingly, middle-aged adults tend to communicate in ways that are different from younger and older people. This can help explain why middle-aged adults are looked to for wisdom and strength when a crisis occurs.

Midlife or middle-aged adults typically range in age from approximately 40–70 years. Middle-aged adults usually have more living relatives than younger or older adults and have many ties to family members above and below their generation. Midlife adults not only have more living family members, but are more engaged with the larger family than older and younger people. Midlife has many balls juggling in the air: most adults are still working and have active social lives and leisure activities. Health concerns related to aging are a new concern for the older end of this group.

Older and younger family members look to the midlife generation for emotional, physical, and financial support at various times. This generation ensures that family relationships are sustained through holiday gatherings and reunions, perhaps providing child care for grandchildren and caring for the older generation. When problems occur, midlife fathers and mothers are first to be called upon and the first to offer help. These activities tend to make them feel good about helping the younger generation.

Midlife adults are generally more emotionally stable and able to see others' needs. This empathy allows midlife adults to see nuances of communication in relationships and to be less likely to be critical or aggressive.

Midlife adults are better at listening and solving problems. When conflict occurs, they are more likely to do nothing, or wait to see things improve rather than yell or use name calling. "When she was angry at the cancer or frustrated because she needed help showering, I didn't try to cheer her up. I just listened," said Martha.

"I would want to cry when the nurse's aides wouldn't help me get her ready to get cleaned up. But, I took a deep breath and got together the supplies and got right into the shower with her," said Stephanie.

Midlife adults are more likely to use constructive rather than destructive strategies with conflict. They understand that treating other people respectfully has practical implications too. "If I blew up, I'd have to apologize eventually. The more people who saw me act like a mad man, the more people I'd have to say I'm sorry to. That would be too much bother," said Greg.

The downside to a calmer communication style is that midlife adults may feel their own needs get ignored. "I was very tired," said Martha, "but I kept on going."

## Getting Your Share So You Can Keep Giving

Some parents found that establishing a routine, along with regular check-ins, helped bring order to the chaos of care and worry when an adult child was seriously ill. "Once we started talking about what they needed and what I could do, things were better," said Dee. "I knew what I could do to help and when I could have time for myself."

Flexibility is key. In the movie *Harry Potter and the Deathly Hallows: Part 2* (Heyman & Yates, 2011), Harry Potter and Hermione Granger talk about the hazards of overplanning:

> Hermione: *"We have to plan! We have to figure out . . ."*
> Harry: *"Hermione! When have our plans ever worked?*
> *We plan, we get there, and all hell breaks loose!"*

Daily routines help. Folding the laundry, washing the car, and going to the gym can make life seem more normal. Go outside. Even if you are only outside long enough to walk to the end of the driveway and get the mail, being outside helps. Having "a good cry" is a time-honored way of feeling better. The release of chemical endorphins when crying relieves stress. Finally, if you have to get angry, get angry at a social injustice, such as a lack of support groups for your child's illness or less-than-excellent health care or doctors making rounds at 5 am to avoid talking to your child and family. This is a productive way to blow off steam and can also release those stress-relieving endorphins. "I said to the nurse: 'Do you know who I am? I am Dr. Smythe, her mother. I want a doctor to check out her pain right now!'" said Judy. It did not matter that Judy Smythe's doctorate was a PhD in English Literature. It got the doctor to order more appropriate medication, and Judy felt much more useful.

## Your Spouse, Partner, or Significant Other

Most midlife adults are married or are part of an intimate relationship. When an adult child's illness takes you away, these loved ones can feel left out, resentful, or angry. Parents have suggested some helpful and not so helpful ways of preserving these relationships during this crisis.

• Remember that your partner may be used to having you all to himself. Jealousy is common when a person's importance is threatened by someone you might love more. Although certainly not attractive, childish behavior is understandable.

- Two unhelpful reactions to your partner's perceived abandonment are:
  - Inappropriate behavior management. Do not say, "Buck up! You're a grown-up! I have to take care of her right now. Don't be a baby." Do not say anything close to such belittling name calling.
  - Being obnoxious. Don't let family relationships be an excuse for spiteful communication. Nothing good ever came from venting your frustrations and anger on those close to you.
- Some examples of helpful reactions to your partner's desire to have you all to herself:
  - Remind your partner how important she is.
  - Have a meal together. Make what you make best—a favorite dinner, baked goods, or perhaps reservations at a favorite restaurant.
  - Consult your partner about decisions you are making.
  - Keep your partner in the loop.
  - Send a special card or e-mail. The message should be similar to "Thank you for being there, for being supportive, for understanding . . . I'm grateful we're a team." Even if partners are not a pillar of support, chances are they know they should be. Thanking your partner can often be the impetus for behavior change.
  - Encourage your partner to keep contact with friends and other family members. In a rare study of fathers of seriously ill children, fathers reported that keeping ties with friends and church and work colleagues helped their resiliency or ability to bounce back from a frightening situation such as a child's illness (Brody & Simmons, 2007).

• You must not accept an abusive reaction to your child's illness. As in all situations with an intimate partner, if you feel threatened, leave and get help.

## Your Other Children

The Smothers Brothers were a popular comedy team in the 1970s. Tommy Smothers would accuse his brother Dick, "Mom always liked you best!" The audience would laugh loudly at the skit every time they played it. This line hits home for every person who was not an only child. Comedy helps us laugh at and cope with things that worry us or make us feel badly about our worthiness.

Sick children's siblings, regardless of their ages, can feel jealous if they think that parents are deferring too much to the sick brother or sister. Temperament affects siblings' reactions. Some siblings become altruistic and others become resentful. Ordinal position affects the reaction of siblings. For example, typically, the oldest child is accustomed to being the boss and the center of attention, the youngest child is used to being the recipient of attention and help, and the middle child just wants to be noticed (or get out of everyone's way when there is strife). Anything that upsets that balance can be perceived as unfair, even if the "baby" has children of his own!

Your other children's reactions can trigger old feelings about your parenting that you thought you had resolved years ago. Parents of ill adult children commonly report feelings of guilt, worry, and trying to make up for shortcomings and regrets. This has been called the "shoulda, woulda, coulda" syndrome.

Happily, the same advice you followed when the children were young can be applied here. Remember when you did something to upset the balance of the household when the children were small, such as bringing home a new baby or going back to work? What was effective then was reassuring them with time and attention. Because adult children should understand your dilemma better than when they were younger, you may find that the energy needed to satisfy them will be less. You may hear, "It's not fair; you spend too much time with her . . . What about me and my kids?" Don't take the bait. Instead remember the three E's:

- Empathize. "I'm sorry you feel that way." "You're right, no one likes this situation." "I understand what you mean." "This is unfair for everyone."
- Engage. "How do you think we could do better with this situation?" "Thank you for helping. This gave me time with you and gave me a real hand."
- Educate. "Let me tell you about what this disease is like." "I want you to remember how much I love you."

Finally, listen to your side of the conversation. Is your part of it all wrapped up in information about your ill child and family? If so, give an overview of their sibling's progress and then ask about their lives and their children's activities.

## Your Child-in-Law

When married adults become seriously ill, the relationship between parents and the child-in-law becomes very important. When a person is married, the next of kin is the spouse. Depending on the age of the married child and the length of the marriage, parents can be sadly surprised to learn that their input is not only not required, but not sought. When difficult or controversial medical decisions need to be made, these interactions can be supportive or destructive.

Public perception of parent–child-in-law relationships during serious illness is not generally positive. The Terri Schiavo case is perhaps the most famous example of parents and a spouse unable to come to a mutually acceptable solution for a young woman who could not speak on her own behalf (Quill, 2005). Both Terri's parents and her spouse thought that their beliefs about life-sustaining treatment were the best way to show love to Terri, but their methods were diametrically different. This sad case brought into question how family is defined and the best way to proceed when sincere disagreements occur.

When married adult children are relatively young, the power imbalance between parents and spouse can create conflict and additional stress. Penny's relationship with her daughter-in-law was tense before her son suddenly became critically ill. During the hospitalization, Penny's name was removed from the list of approved visitors in the intensive care unit. "When I found out, I told his wife that I was there when he came into this world, and I will be there when he leaves," said Penny. "Even now, when I think about how we couldn't stand to be in the same room when Jim was so sick, I feel horrible." Penny felt highly threatened by being separated from her son. Yet, her reaction endangered her future relationship with her daughter-in-law and grandchildren. This is understandable. Parents tend to feel they have more to gain and lose in their relationship with their adult children. This is called the Intergenerational Stake

Hypothesis. Recognizing this unbalanced social investment can be a first step as parents work to create a climate of trust and support (Wrzus, Wagner, Baumert, Neyer, & Lang, 2011).

Research has shown that secure attachment between parents and adult children and their spouses is associated with collaborating and compromising when serious life events occur. A dismissive or preoccupied parental attitude often results in more indirect infighting (LaValley & Guerrero, 2012). As Julie said, "It kind of depends [on] how you got along before he got sick."

Bonnie says this was her "hard-won lesson." She learned to accept that her daughter's husband came first, even when she

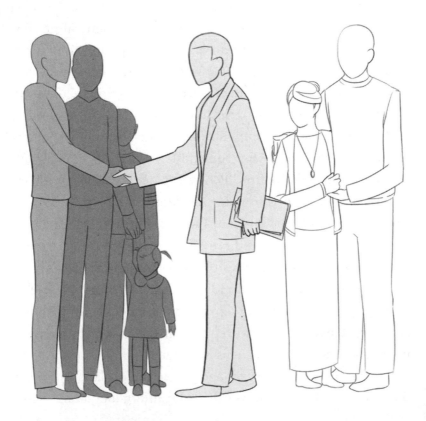

perceived the marriage was poor. She thinks that she is perceived as being more supportive when she is agreeable to her daughter and son-in-law's decisions.

Parents may give support to children-in-law because it is support directed to their child. "I split the household duties with my son-in-law," said Julie. "It helped my daughter's recovery."

A climate of trust and the relationship's history seem to affect the parent–child-in-law relationship when adult children are seriously ill. "She is part of our family and will be for a long time. I knew that. I was the more mature person in this situation and so I reached out," said Marge. "I do it for my son and our entire family."

## Your Friends

More experts than can be listed here recognize that friends who offer emotional support decrease stress. When serious illness occurs, not all friends stick around. Some friends can't cope with being close to illness or don't know what to say. A sick child can represent a real threat to another parent. A friend may have an adult child who is the same age or an adult child who has a chronic illness that may take the person's life early (Brown, 2010). The more vulnerable a parent-friend feels, the more likely she will become distant. "Some of my friends acted like what [my daughter] had was contagious," said Stephanie. "I'm lonely and tired, and my friends don't have a clue."

"You choose who you tell," said Danielle.

Some friends will offer to help and then not show, and others will help in unemotional ways, such as bringing a meal or raking leaves, but don't want to be alone with you or your ill adult child. "My sister is my best friend. When Sean was sick, she was a good listener, but she was emotionally closed," said Susan. "She was happiest when I gave her a job to do like grocery shopping."

Taking into account the fear that losing a child represents, it may be more amazing that one or two good friends stick it out. Parents who have been through this are unanimous in their advice.

"Use the network you've built over the years. Those connections will keep you sane," said Anne.

"You learn to find help. Try not to feel resentful and say, 'Well, now I know who my friends are.' Take support when it is offered," said Danielle.

If your adult child has cancer and you feel as though you have no friends or family members who understand what you are going through, the 4th Angel program may be able to help. The 4th Angel is a patient and caregiver mentoring program that offers free confidential support from someone who has made the same journey. More information about 4th Angel is found in this chapter's "By the Way…" section.

## Have We Forgotten Anyone?

Aunts and uncles and in-laws and stepfamilies are sometimes called the "forgotten kin" (Milardo, 2010). They can be important sources of support. These relationships can serve as intergenerational buffers. They understand the family culture and nuances of family interaction because they are part of the family history. If you live out of town, family members can be a source of information and crisis assistance (Mazanec, Daly, Ferrell, & Prince-Paul, 2011). Family members can be helpful when you think you caused the illness, such as when a genetic link is discovered (Raveis & Pretter, 2005; Zapka, Fisher, Lemon, Clemow, & Fletcher, 2006). Family members can help diminish guilt because they understand you in ways that other friends may not. Sometimes it seems easier to ask family members for help.

"Ask family for help without apology," said Pat. "What is the worst that can happen? They will turn you down. What is the best that can happen? You and your immediate family will get some respite and new ideas."

## If I Have to Tell One More Person

"I was telling the same story over and over again," said Katherine. "I was tired of hearing my own voice and wondered if I was remembering everything Jack asked me to tell."

Keeping family and friends informed about your adult child's illness can be a daunting task. As a parent of a very ill adult child, you may be asked to help keep family and some friends up to date. The list can be pretty long, and the need to tell can be very frequent, especially during acute periods of illness and treatment. You don't have the time, the memory, or the inclination to make multiple phone calls every week. If you forget an important person (or a person who thinks he's important), you risk closing off a potential source of support, or worse, inadvertently hurting the feelings of a truly important person.

There is an answer: social media. *Social media* is a broad term that describes using the Internet to communicate with large numbers of people. Social media is all about connecting people to one another. Social media is also called social networking and includes technology such as e-mail, Facebook, blogs, Twitter, and Google+. Social media requires access to a computer, tablet, or smartphone.

Happily, most social media platforms are easy to use and have help built in to the program. You don't have to be a computer expert to quickly learn how to use social media to communicate with large groups of people. Katrina said it well: "Social media helped me tell what was going on to friends and family without retelling. Sarah and her husband and children and my husband and I were amazed with how much support and help we got."

Before using social media, a few important caveats need to be mentioned.

- A comment or posting on social media, like any form of Internet communication, never goes away. Great care needs to be taken with who you are telling information and what information you are sharing. You cannot take back hurtful or humiliating comments.
- Don't assume you are considered the primary source of information. The news about your adult child's illness and treatment is not your news to tell. Ask permission to keep family and friends up to date on his progress. You are his parent and might think you should be able to share information about your child, but he is a grown-up and you should not tell without permission.
- Make sure you know who your child wants to keep informed.

Don't send out a broadcast to everyone both of you know. Be discriminate.

- It's a good idea to ask permission if you want to share personal information about your adult child's illness with your friends. You do deserve to have support for yourself, but you may want to consider talking about how the illness is affecting you, and go easy on the intimate details about your child.
- If you think that a topic might cause your child embarrassment, ask yourself: Would it be okay if the people at church heard about it . . . from the pulpit? If the answer is no, then reconsider telling anyone. This includes all comments about vomiting, diarrhea, and things said while on painkillers.

## Loretta's Story

After some frank conversations with her husband and other children, Loretta decided to stay on the schedule with Lori and her family that had worked so well. The family seemed to cope better during the weeks Lori had chemotherapy if Loretta was there to keep the household running smoothly. Loretta talked to her book club about her dilemma and found most of her friends very eager to help. Some brought dinner to Loretta's husband and some invited him over for cards or a movie. Today, he jokes about his wife's "army" who brought him not just food and fun, but a respite from loneliness.

One result of the discussions with her grandchildren was the discovery of the social media tool, Skype. With the help of her son-in-law and grandson, Lori and her siblings, as well as all her grandchildren, visit each week on their home computers.

# Conclusion

The threat of families breaking apart during the crisis of serious illness is very real. The support of friends is also at risk when it seems as though parents are diverting too much time to their ill child. Middle-aged parents, because of their life experiences and willingness to hold relationships together, are in an excellent position to sustain support for themselves and the other important people in their lives.

# References

Birditt, K.S., & Fingerman, K.L. (2005). Do we get better at picking our battles? Age group differences in descriptions of behavioral reactions to interpersonal tensions. *Journals of Gerontology: Series B Psychological Sciences and Social Sciences, 60B*, 121–128. doi:10.1093/geronb/60.3.P121

Brody, A.C., & Simmons, L. (2007). Family resiliency during childhood cancer: The father's perspective. *Journal of Pediatric Oncology Nursing, 24*, 152–165. doi:10.1177/1043454206298844

Brown, H. (2010, August 16). Coping with crises close to someone else's heart. *New York Times*. Retrieved from http://www.nytimes.com/2010/08/17/health/views/17essa.html

Fingerman, K.L., & Birditt, K.S. (2003). Do age differences in close and problematic family ties reflect the pool of available relatives? *Journals of Gerontology: Series B Psychological Sciences and Social Sciences, 58B*, 80–87. doi:10.1093/geronb/58.2.P80

Fingerman, K.L., Nussbaum, J., & Birditt, K.S. (2004). Keeping all five balls in the air: Juggling family communication at midlife. In A.L. Vangelisti (Ed.), *Handbook of family communication* (pp. 135–152). Mahwah, NJ: Lawrence Erlbaum Associates.

Heyman, D. (Producer), & Yates, D. (Director). (2011). *Harry Potter and the deathly hallows: Part 2* [Motion picture]. United States: Warner Brothers.

LaValley, A.G., & Guerrero, L.K. (2012). Perceptions of conflict behavior and relational satisfaction in adult parent-child relationships: A dyadic analysis from an attachment perspective. *Communication Research, 39*, 48–78. doi:10.1177/0093650210391655

Mazanec, P.M., Daly, B.J., Ferrell, B.R., & Prince-Paul, M. (2011). Lack of communication and control: Experiences of distance caregivers of parents with advanced cancer. *Oncology Nursing Forum, 38,* 307 313. doi:10.1188/11.ONF.307-313

Milardo, R.M. (2010). *The forgotten kin.* New York, NY: Cambridge University Press.

Miller-Day, M.A. (2004). *Communication among grandmothers, mothers and adult daughters: A qualitative study of maternal relationships.* Mahwah, NJ: Lawrence Erlbaum Associates.

Quill, T.E. (2005). Terri Schiavo—A tragedy compounded. *New England Journal of Medicine, 352,* 1630–1633. doi:10.1056/NEJMp058062

Raveis, V.H., & Pretter, S. (2005). Existential plight of adult daughters following their mother's breast cancer diagnosis. *Psycho-Oncology, 14,* 49–60. doi:10.1002/pon.819

Wrzus, C., Wagner, J., Baumert, A., Neyer, F.J., & Lang, F.R. (2011). Adult parent-child relationships through the lens of social relations analyses: Prosocial personality and reciprocity of support. *European Journal of Personality, 25,* 133–145. doi:10.1002/per.802

Zapka, J., Fisher, G., Lemon, S., Clemow, L., & Fletcher, K. (2006). Relationship and distress in relatives of breast cancer patients. *Families, Systems and Health: The Journal of Collaborative Family Healthcare, 24,* 198–212. doi:10.1037/1091-7527.24.2.198

## By the Way...

- Don't be hard on yourself. Your reaction can be different from one day to the next or within the same day depending on the time of day or new information.
- The Golden Rule applies even more than usual because if you blow up to a group, the number of "I'm sorrys" can be daunting.
- Blow off steam productively.
- CaringBridge is a free social media site (www.caringbridge.org) that allows you or your adult child to develop a personalized Web page and blog about your adult child's illness experiences. Access to this Web site is controlled; friends and family are invited to view the site. Friends and family can respond to entries.
- Lotsa Helping Hands (www.lotsahelpinghands.com) is a free site that will help you build a community of friends and family to organize help and support. For example, you can create a calendar with names of people who are bringing dinners to your adult child's family each day. You can give medical status updates. Lotsa Helping Hands also provides a monthly webinar.
- The 4th Angel Patient and Caregiver Mentoring Program (www.4thangel.org) is an important part of the Scott Hamilton CARES initiative. A 4th Angel is someone who has been a patient with cancer or caregiver for a person with cancer. 4th Angel offers free, confidential mentoring support by volunteer mentors through its Web site, by telephone (216-445-8734 or 866-520-3197), or via e-mail (4thangel@ccf.org).
- The "Caregiving" page on the Centers for Medicare and Medicaid Services (www.medicare.gov/caregivers) provides multiple sources of assistance to family caregivers. Instructions for obtaining government financial and health benefits are included on the site.
- Thousands of social media sites are available; some may offer support specific to your circumstances. To find these sites, you can use popular search engines, such as Google, Yahoo, or Bing, or the search box located on your browser's homepage. Some examples of keyword searches are "social media for chronic illness," "lung cancer online support groups," and "diabetes blogs." You may need to adjust your search terms to find the group that is right for you, especially if the search returns too many or too few Web sites.

# CHAPTER 3

# CARING FOR YOUR CHILD:
# Physical Care

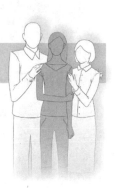

*I walked a mile with Sorrow,*
*And ne'er a word said she;*
*But, oh! The things I learned from her,*
*When Sorrow walked with me.*

—Robert Browning Hamilton

## Annette's Story

While in law school and only 23 years old, Sophia was diagnosed with ovarian cancer. The first treatment for her cancer was extensive surgery. On the outside, this surgery left her with a scar down the center of her abdomen stretching from the bottom of her breast bone to the top of her pubic bone. Internally, the surgery resulted in removing the cancer along with her reproductive organs and pieces of her colon, liver, spleen, and diaphragm. It was major surgery that required four days in intensive care and about a month in the hospital. Her mother, Annette, was by her side.

The very night after surgery, Annette, who was a nurse, noticed the pain medication wasn't working. Sophia was receiving pain medication through an epidural catheter. This puts the medication directly into the spine, a method used often and successfully for women in labor. Sophia's pain, which should have been about a 1 or 2 on a 0–10 scale, where 10 is "the worst pain imaginable," was 10–12! She was getting more and more upset whenever Annette went back to see her during posted visiting hours. Annette was forced out of the mother role and spoke "nurse to nurse" with the nurse caring for Sophia. Eventually they determined that the epidural catheter was not in the correct position; the pain medication was not being delivered to the proper place to work effectively. The problem was corrected, but Sophia became even more insistent that Annette stay with her. It would not be the last time she had to speak up on her daughter's behalf.

Once out of the hospital, Sophia returned to law school about 500 miles from Annette's home in Texas. "She made the decision that she wanted to stay in school in Oklahoma, and I think that it was the best decision she ever made," said Annette. It was not easy, but nothing about having a seriously ill child was easy.

Sophia had about a four-month disease-free remission. This was much too short, and she needed chemotherapy. With guidance from her physicians, Annette and Sophia researched her treatment options. Learning about what Sophia's treatment options were, finding clinical trials she might be eligible for, and financing her care required skill and time. Annette recalls, "That was a full-time job, and I think it pulled us together."

Eventually, Sophia was enrolled in a clinical trial conducted at the National Cancer Institute using what at the time was a novel chemotherapy drug, bevacizumab. "It was very hopeful," Annette says of that time. This drug and others would keep her ovarian cancer more or less under control for more than five years.

Although five years was also much too short of a time, Sophia's life was not all about the cancer. She also had the time to finish law school, work for the State Department of Corrections reviewing death penalty cases, and get married. She and Justin were married for two years before she died. Annette and Thomas had been her parents for almost 29 years, more than half of their lives, when Sophia died.

The struggles with a seriously ill child are multifaceted, but not the least is how to physically care for a beloved adult child. It is impossible to overstate the importance of physical care. At the end of her life, Sophia had her loved ones around her in her own home. The burden of care through rehabilitation and later cancer treatment fell on Annette. Sophia was always hopeful for a cure or long-term remission, but at the end of her life, hospice care in her home was appropriate. Never underestimate the power of physical care.

The importance of physical care has been recognized by many, including Joseph Cardinal Bernardin in his 1997 book *The Gift of Peace*: "Make sure that you pray when you're well because when you're real sick, you probably won't" (p. 67). He recognized that if you are overwhelmed with pain or nausea and vomiting, as he experienced with his cancer, you cannot properly pray. Sure, you may be saying, "Oh my God, help me," but it is a plea, not a spiritual revelation.

Along with the physical care needs, touch is very important. When someone is seriously ill, touch is often associated with pain. It might be the pain of having blood drawn, surgery, or other medical procedures. Sometimes, a person will be more sensitive to touch when something hurts. However, touching someone you love is always a good thing to do. There are very few, if any, circumstances when touch would be the wrong thing to do. One woman recalled that after her surgery for breast cancer, it was her mother who stepped into the shower with her to help handle the drains and cleanse the body parts she couldn't reach. Another woman recalls her mother holding her in bed when her husband left her after hearing that she was diagnosed with multiple sclerosis. Touch is healing and always important.

Among all the care needs of people who are ill, physical needs usually are first. As in Sophia's first night after her surgery, her physical pain was not controlled. At that time, nothing else mattered. It is true that often emotional, spiritual, and

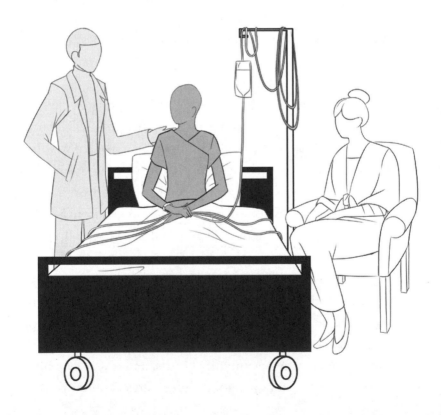

financial needs compound physical ailments. They are all important and discussed elsewhere in this book. But it is difficult, if not impossible, to concentrate on strengthening these without physical care. In this chapter, select basic physical needs will be discussed along with strategies to meet them. These needs have been identified repeatedly by ill adults and their families as areas of concern. They are the needs to

- Breathe easily
- Have food and water
- Be free from pain
- Overcome fatigue.

Comfort is more than just the absence of physical pain. Being comfortable may be breathing easier. It may be choosing to tolerate some physical pain because the side effects of the medication are undesirable. It is important for parents to talk to their children and know what their priorities are. What do they want? This chapter will help you understand these needs and how they relate to serious illness and medical treatments. Finally, it will give you some ideas of ways that you can help meet these needs.

## The Need to Breathe Easily

Very ill people often say, "The worst thing is when I can't catch my breath." The need to breathe easily is important for good quality of life. Studies have shown that it ranks above the need to be free from pain. The purpose of breathing is to inhale oxygen and exhale carbon dioxide. When a person is well, this process is largely unconscious.

Oxygen is required to sustain life. The oxygen that we breathe in is transported by the blood to every living cell in the body. Along with other waste products of cellular metabolism, carbon dioxide is taken by the blood from every cell back to the lungs and removed from the body during exhalation. The cardiac and respiratory systems work together to meet the body's need for oxygen and are helped by chemical and nervous system responses.

## Abnormalities Related to Serious Illness

*Dyspnea* is a subjective sensation of difficult or uncomfortable breathing. It is also called shortness of breath, and it is normal with exercise or excitement. But dyspnea is more than that. It is a problem when it occurs without any relation to activity or exercise because of disease or injury. It is distressful to the patient and caregivers. As a man with lung cancer described, "The tightness in my chest and the difficulty I have in catching my breath is like when I was well and had just finished running a marathon. At the end of the run, I felt that I could not possibly go any further. I was short of breath and felt exhausted. Now, I feel like that all the time. It never stops. There is no relief."

The exact mechanism of dyspnea is not completely understood and cannot be accurately measured. Although the amount of oxygen in the blood can be measured, this does not correlate to how well a person feels they are breathing. A person may report no trouble breathing when his blood has very low oxygen levels, whereas another person may report very difficult breathing although his oxygen levels are normal. The only reliable indicator for dyspnea or breathlessness, like pain, is self-report.

Breathing difficulties can manifest with other symptoms. These include pain, fatigue, coughing, and wheezing. Other signs of breathing difficulties include paleness, cyanosis or a blue tinge around the lips or the nail beds, labored breathing using many or all of the chest and neck muscles, and being unable to breathe unless sitting upright.

Many conditions can affect breathing. These include heart problems, lung problems, and blood disorders, particularly anemia. Pregnancy, musculoskeletal abnormalities, neurologic diseases, and infections can detrimentally affect breathing. Lifestyle factors such as cigarette smoking, obesity, alcohol and drug abuse, lack of exercise, and stress all can add to breathing difficulties. Environmental exposure to pollution and asbestos may also make breathing more difficult.

## Medical Management

Testing the adequacy of breathing may be done by simple measurements of heart and respiratory rates per minute, or checking oxygen saturation or the amount of oxygen on the red blood cells, with a sensor on the fingertip or measuring the amount of oxygen in a blood sample. Tests can also be more sophisticated when looking for a diagnosis and may include x-rays, scans, or biopsies.

Treating dyspnea should start with treating the underlying cause if possible. When the underlying cause cannot be treated effectively, often several interventions may be used together to make breathing easier. Treatment options with their advantages and disadvantages should be discussed with a physician. Questions must be answered satisfactorily and in a way that can be understood. Adults always have the right to refuse a treatment that they consider unacceptable. Some medical treatments for dyspnea include the following.

- Incentive spirometry uses a measured tube with a mouthpiece through which a person inhales slowly and deeply, trying to keep a freely moving colored ball floating as long as possible. This promotes deep breathing and fills the lungs with air.

- Oxygen can be given by a nasal cannula, which is a simple tube that is inserted into the nose or by a mask that covers the mouth and nose.

- Artificial airways, chest tubes, and ventilators are sophisticated and complex medical interventions to help with breathing.

- Comfort medications may include opioids, narcotics, anti-anxiety medications, sedatives, or a combination of these. These are given to relax muscles and to decrease anxiety, which will make breathing easier. Other pharmacologic interventions or medications that may be prescribed to ease breathing are bronchodilators to relax smooth muscles of the respiratory tract and relieve spasm or diuretics to decrease congestion and fluid overload.

- Suctioning can remove secretions that may be blocking airways and interfering with breathing.

- Chest physiotherapy uses a variety of positions and compressions to help remove secretions.

- Blood transfusion can be given for anemia.

## How to Help

Along with the prescribed medical treatments, some lifestyle interventions can be used to help ease breathing.

- Often, prioritizing what activities are most important is necessary. Choices may have to be made about what to spend energy on and what must either be denied or delayed for another day.
- Smoking cessation, healthy eating, weight reduction, appropriate exercise, and balancing of rest, exercise, and activity may also be considered if appropriate.
- Increasing ambient airflow directed at the face or nose with a fan or humidifier can help.
- Pursed-lip breathing slows respirations.
- Cooler room temperatures will keep your loved one more comfortable.
- Techniques such as using a chair when bathing, keeping frequently used objects close by, and sitting in a recliner will help conserve energy.
- Elevating the head of the bed or using forward/upward positioning with the bedside table and pillows may be helpful.
- Music can create a calm room environment.
- Relaxation techniques and stress reduction are helpful (see Appendix).

## The Need to Have Food and Water

In our culture, food is important for more than just survival. We often use food as a way of showing that we care for someone. It plays a big part in our social events and adds routine to the day. We take pleasure in eating and associate it with feeling better or living longer. Common worries when someone is ill and not eating are that they will suffer and starve or that dehydration makes people sick. Often we hear, "If she doesn't eat, she will die sooner"; "I want him to get stronger"; and "I want to provide the best care for him." These comments may or may not be realistic within the circumstances of the illness.

## Abnormalities Related to Serious Illness

*Anorexia* refers to a loss of appetite that may be associated with an advanced illness or side effects from treatments such as chemotherapy. This does not refer to the eating disorder, anorexia nervosa. In late-stage cancers, anorexia is reported to be as high as 70%–80% and can lead to weight loss and malnutrition. Factors that may lead to a decreased appetite include nausea and vomiting, constipation, pain, weakness and fatigue, side effects of chemotherapy or other medications, or mouth sores and other dental problems. Some diseases associated with nausea and vomiting and a decreased appetite are partial or complete bowel obstruction, infections, cancer, fear or anxiety, liver failure, or kidney failure.

## Medical Management

Medical treatments that might improve appetite and eating include the following.

• Medications such as corticosteroids for short-term treatment or some hormones can be used to stimulate the appetite.

• Nausea and vomiting should be treated if they are problematic. The medications prescribed will depend on the cause of nausea and vomiting and when they occur. Treatment is dictated by treating the presumed cause if feasible. Try interventions that have worked in the past. Many different categories of medications are available by prescription for nausea and vomiting. Often, a combination is most helpful. Some trial and error may be involved before the best combination is found. Everyone is different, and timing is key.

- Individualized dietary counseling and meeting with a dietitian to discuss preparing foods will help make them more nutritious and appealing.

- Artificial nutrition and hydration, also called ANH or medically administered nutrition and hydration or tube feeding, is a medical intervention that some patients need if they cannot consume adequate nutrition by mouth. Before beginning a complex treatment like this, a discussion with the physician is very important so that the expected benefits, advantages and disadvantages, and potential side effects are clearly understood. Generally, ANH is given through a feeding using the intestinal tract in which a tube is placed either through the nose to the stomach or inserted through a small incision directly into the abdominal wall to the stomach or small intestine. ANH may also be given using the intravenous route.

ANH may benefit those who cannot swallow during an acute event or for a short time but are expected to regain the ability to swallow, those who are receiving intensive treatment such as radiation therapy for head and neck cancer, people with a gastrointestinal obstruction, and patients who are recovering from injury or stroke. ANH may be more harmful than beneficial when given to someone whose inability to maintain nutrition is because of a chronic, debilitating, life-limiting disease; the dying process; advanced dementia; or end-stage kidney failure. These are difficult decisions and should be made only after full informed-consent discussions.

The benefits and burdens must always be considered. That is, will ANH help the person feel better or get well? Or will it cause more suffering and prolong the inevitable? ANH supplies nutrition and fluid artificially. Side effects can include painful swelling under the skin, stomach distention, or diarrhea for those whose systems are shutting down during the end of life.

To compare and contrast the various considerations with ANH, reflect on the similarities and differences in the following two situations. First is a 50-year-old man who had a brain tumor that only affected his ability to swallow. He was recovering nicely after surgery and chose to use a feeding tube until he could swallow again. When he was again able to swallow, the feeding tube was removed.

In another case, a 47-year-old woman suffering from early and severe-onset dementia had already lost her decision-making capacity and was losing the ability to swallow. When this happened, her family, on her behalf, decided that a feeding tube would not be placed. They would continue to help her eat and drink as she was able, but her dementia was a terminal illness and they would not risk further complications with a medical procedure. The benefits did not outweigh the risks in their estimation. The absence of a feeding tube did not alter the course of the disease, nor would its insertion have altered the disease. She continued to be well cared for and comfortable until she died of her dementia.

## How to Help

There are many ways to help someone who is having difficulty eating and drinking. Generally, nagging, insisting, demanding, and arguing are not those ways. Helpful interventions may include:

- Serving small, frequent meals. Avoid sweet, salty, fatty, and spicy foods unless these taste good to the person eating. Offer favorite foods in small amounts. Encourage the person to eat slowly. Bland, cold, or room-temperature food is often best tolerated.
- Offering food during "good hours" when energy is high and pain is low.
- Controlling odor around meal preparation and serving.
- Giving oral care before and after meals and after each episode of vomiting.
- Limiting fluids with meals until eating is done. An exception might be having wine or another alcoholic drink before meals, particularly if that is an enjoyed habit.
- Pureeing foods if swallowing is difficult. Use liquid meals or supplements to give the most calories and nutrients in the simplest, easiest-to-take form.
- Giving ice chips, Popsicles®, or sips of favorite beverages to relieve dry mouth. Mouth care with moistened swabs may also help.
- Assisting or feeding by hand if necessary. This is a way to be close and helpful.
- Preparing the proper social setting for meals and a pleasing presentation of meals.

## The Need to Be Free From Pain

Pain is "whatever the experiencing person says it is and existing whenever he says it does," said pain expert Margo McCaffery

40 years ago (Mann & Carr, 2006, pp. 1–2). Pain is subjective. There is no objective test that can measure it. A person's report of pain must be believed.

Any stimulation that can cause damage to skin or tissue, such as a sharp or blunt object, heat, or chemicals, can result in pain. *Acute pain* is a warning that something is wrong and usually persists less than three months. *Chronic pain* is defined primarily by duration, persisting for weeks, months, or years, and cannot usually be fully relieved by standard pain medications. People who suffer with chronic pain are unlikely to show behavioral changes because they have adapted to their level of pain. This is not the same as having no pain.

People react differently to pain; some are dramatic, some are stoic, and some look just fine. Both acute and chronic pains require treatment. Remember that pain is subjective. If the ill person says he is in pain, believe it.

People may hold many false beliefs about pain. These often prejudice them against a person who complains of pain or makes them doubt that person. The following are some of the more common myths about pain.

- Drug abusers and alcoholics overreact to discomforts.
- People with minor illnesses have less pain than those with severe illnesses.
- Using analgesics regularly will lead to drug addiction.
- The amount of tissue damage in an injury accurately indicates the pain intensity.
- Psychological pain is not real.
- Chronic pain is psychological.
- You should expect to have pain in a hospital.
- You should have no pain in a hospital.

- People who cannot communicate do not feel pain; this includes the very young, the very old, those with mental disorders, or those who cannot speak English.

## Abnormalities Related to Serious Illness

The transmission and perception of pain is a complex process. This process includes:

- Pain receptors are present throughout the body in varying concentrations. The skin, joints, and arterial walls have large numbers, the gut and muscle have fewer, and the brain has none.
- Chemicals called neurotransmitters are released by injured tissue and initiate the firing of nerve cells to transmit pain. Neurotransmitters start a chain reaction that will produce inflammation, causing the surrounding area to become increasingly painful.
- Nerve fibers transmit the sensation of pain from the painful sites through the spinal cord traveling to the brain. In the brain, pain is recognized, located, and acted upon.
- Additional neurotransmitters are released by the brain that can positively affect the pain response. For example, endorphins act directly on the central nervous system to reduce the pain experience.
- If pain becomes chronic, that is, persisting for more than three months, other areas of the brain become involved and influence the perception of pain. This is very individualized but helps explain how pain is influenced by past pain experiences. Evidence also suggests that in chronic pain, how an individual responds to and what is believed about pain impact quality of life more than pain intensity (Mann & Carr, 2006).

## Medical Management

Whenever possible, the underlying cause of pain should be treated. When the underlying cause cannot be treated effectively, many pharmacologic and nonpharmacologic interventions are available. Often a combination of interventions works best, but it may take some trial and error to determine which is best for a person. These combinations take advantage of what is understood about the perception and transmission of pain described in the previous section. The active ingredients in pain medications or analgesics attempt to disrupt the pain sensation at several different points.

Generally, medications that are prescribed for pain are either nonopioid analgesics or opioid analgesics. Nonopioid analgesics may be bought over the counter or require a prescription.

Some nonopioid analgesics include acetaminophen (Tylenol®), aspirin, ibuprofen (Motrin®), naproxen (Naprosyn®), and celecoxib (Celebrex®). Although these medications have different actions, they generally influence pain peripherally, that is, outside the brain and spinal cord. The side effects can be serious, and medications should be taken only as directed.

Opioid analgesics, also sometimes called narcotics, require a prescription. They generally act centrally, in the brain, to affect perceptions and reactions to pain. Some are combination medications such as Vicodin®, which has the opioid hydrocodone plus the nonopioid acetaminophen in it. It has the advantage of both medications in a single pill, but people who take combination medications must also be aware of the side effects of the individual ingredients. For example, acetaminophen can cause severe, irreversible liver damage if taken in high doses. People on Vicodin should be warned to avoid taking additional acetaminophen when taking this drug. Straight opioids are not used in combination, such as morphine and oxycodone. As always, these medications have side effects, but these should be distinguished from expected reactions. For example, when first taking an opioid such as morphine, a person may experience pain relief with some drowsiness and nausea. These reactions are expected and can be controlled with other medications if necessary and eventually a tolerance is developed. They are not allergic reactions, as some mistakenly believe.

Pain medications come in a variety of formulas for administering them, such as pills and liquids for oral ingestion, injections for intravenous or subcutaneous administration, patches in which the medication is absorbed through the skin, and suppositories for rectal administration. The easiest route for the person and the qualities of the pain itself will dictate which formula to use.

Medication formulas also vary in regard to release of active ingredients. Sustained release and instant release formulas are both available in some medications. They are often both prescribed for constant pain. The sustained release formula will be given regularly around the clock, and the instant release formula will be used for unexpected or increased pain, also known as breakthrough pain.

## How to Help

There are many ways the medical management of pain can be supplemented. These measures will help provide relief, but they do not cure the pain. So they, just like the medications, work best if repeated regularly. Not all of these will work for everyone, but you can try different approaches to see what is best.

One reliable source for information about nontraditional or nonpharmacologic pain relief methods is the National Center for Complementary and Alternative Medicine (http://nccam.nih.gov). It is a division of the National Institutes of Health whose mission is to explore complementary and alternative healing practices in the context of rigorous science, train complementary and alternative medicine researchers, and disseminate authoritative information to the public and professionals. For example, research has shown that touch, heat, or cold can be used successfully to treat pain (see Appendix).

Finally, a sense of humor may help distract people from their pain and reduce the stress in a difficult situation for all involved. Here are a few favorite lines to think about.

> *If there's one thing I know, it's that God loves a good joke.*
>
> —Hugh Elliott

> *I'm not funny. What I am is brave.*
>
> —Lucille Ball

> *I am thankful for laughter, except when milk comes out of my nose.*
>
> —Woody Allen

## The Need to Overcome Fatigue

"Why am I so tired all the time? I can't do anything. Why won't God make me better?" were Rose's words to her family when she became terminally ill with metastatic colon cancer. There were no answers. People often lack the energy, words, or language that would make doctors, nurses, and others understand just how tired they feel. This bone-deep tiredness, also known as fatigue, is a subjective feeling of exhaustion not relieved by rest. It severely impairs one's quality of life. Because no one says, "I'm fatigued," you must listen for other words that tell you of their fatigue. These words include "tired," "exhausted," "can't get off the couch," "I don't feel like doing anything today . . . or yesterday . . . or the day before." Fatigue is more than not getting enough sleep, although that may be a component of it.

## Abnormalities Related to Serious Illness

Fatigue may be related to disease, treatment, or psychological stressors. Causes include cancer, coronary artery disease, chronic fatigue syndrome, chronic obstructive pulmonary disease, end-stage renal disease, HIV/AIDS, multiple sclerosis, Parkinson disease, and other serious illnesses.

Many of the fatigue studies have been conducted on people with cancer. *Fatigue* is defined as "a distressing, persistent, subjective sense of physical, emotional, and/or cognitive tiredness or exhaustion related to cancer or cancer treatment that is not proportional to recent activity and interferes with usual functioning" (National Comprehensive Cancer Network, 2011). It is the most common symptom reported by patients with cancer during treatment. An estimated 80%–100% of people with cancer experience fatigue. Fatigue may be related directly to the cancer or its treatment and may continue for years after treatment is completed. It may occur as an isolated symptom or as one element in a cluster of symptoms such as pain, depression, sleep disturbance, and anemia.

## Medical Management

The medical management of fatigue is, once again, directed at the underlying cause whenever possible. Medications that may be prescribed include steroids, stimulants, antidepressants, and erythropoietin or red blood cell growth factor. A closer look at all medications being taken may allow some to be decreased or stopped if they are contributing to fatigue. These may include sedatives, hypnotics, analgesics, antiemetics, or antihistamines. If anemia is contributing to fatigue, a blood transfusion may be prescribed.

## How to Help

The basis for helping relieve fatigue is to promote rest, energy conservation, and restoration. Maintaining a routine and getting some fresh air each day have been shown to help. Something (researchers are not sure exactly what) is restorative about the outdoors and nature.

Regular exercise has been shown to be beneficial in relieving fatigue and improving quality of life. This may be home-based exercise or a more structured, supervised exercise program (Wanchai, Armer, & Stewart, 2011).

Although fatigue is not only about getting enough sleep, promoting restful sleep may help decrease fatigue. Ways to promote sleep include:

• Maintaining a regular bedtime and wake-up schedule
• Eliminating naps unless they are a routine part of a schedule
• Going to bed when sleepy
• Using warm bath and relaxation techniques (see Appendix).

Other interventions include the following.

- If the person is unable to fall asleep within 20–30 minutes, suggest getting out of bed and doing some quiet activity until he or she is sleepy enough to go back to bed.
- Earplugs and eyeshades may be helpful.
- Suggest sleeping where the person sleeps best.
- Keep noise to a minimum, and use white noise or soft music to mask noise if necessary.
- Set room temperature to the person's preference.
- Encourage the person to limit alcohol, caffeine, and nicotine in late afternoon and evening.
- Offer carbohydrates or milk as a light snack before bedtime; avoid serving heavy meals three hours before bedtime.
- Remind the person to decrease fluids two to four hours before sleep.
- Elevate the head of the bed and use pillows as preferred.
- Offer analgesics 30 minutes before bed to ease pain.
- Encourage the person to balance exercise and rest and to avoid vigorous exercise within two hours of bedtime.
- Help the person to avoid using the bed for non-sleep activity, except sex.

# The Whole Person

The needs to breathe easily, have food and water, be free from pain, and overcome fatigue are needs that everyone has that should be met. Physical needs can be overwhelming. As one mother declared, her role was to look at the whole person, her son, and make sure his needs were met. "I need to make sure that Jim, the person, is at the center of anything that is planned, at the center of any care that is given. He is not met-astatic testicular cancer but he is Jim with testicular cancer."

Sometimes the whole person is best remembered with a sense of humor. For example, Jim's art major roommate decorated his bald head with washable markers, declaring a masterpiece. It was a little harder for Jim's mother when she saw him in the hospital after major surgery, "with more tubes than orifices."

One afternoon he greeted her with two tears rolling down the face she had loved for 22 years. "You have to help me," he whispered.

While she was away, Jim had a nasogastric tube, a flexible plastic tube, put into his nose and threaded into his stomach. This was to help with his postoperative nausea, vomiting, and gas. The nasogastric tube was a way to relieve the gas, disten-tion, and increasing pressure and size of his abdomen. But he could not tolerate it. It made him gag uncontrollably. Jim's mom insisted it be removed. And it was. It took a little longer, but eventually his gastrointestinal system started working on its own and in the right direction to relieve his nausea, vom-iting, and gas.

When looking at the whole person, a person's sexuality should not be denied or ignored. During illness, an adult's needs related to sexuality may be closely related to feelings and fears about attractiveness and fertility. The past discussions the parent and child have had in these areas will influence how to best approach this area of need. This may not be an area that a parent can help with as much as referring to another adult or professional with whom your child may feel comfortable dis-cussing these issues.

As one mother related, when her 28-year-old son was diagnosed with non-Hodgkin lymphoma and about to start chemotherapy, she asked him and his doctor about fertility. Emphasizing by pointing to an invisible mark on the table, she said, "I wanted to know about future grandchildren."

Once she brought up the subject, her son was referred to a counselor and banked his sperm. This was done quickly so that treatment would not be unnecessarily delayed. She is content with this outcome. "Even today, five years after the treatment, I continue to pay the annual bill for the sperm bank. And I pay it happily," she adds.

Issues of sexuality and fertility can be more complex than this example. Bringing them into the open and then connecting with experts may be the biggest help a parent can give in this area. Always remember the whole person. Remember that the person going through the disease and treatment is more than their disease and treatment.

## Annette's Story

Having a seriously ill child, no matter the age of the child, is difficult. Parents and their children have a bond that is almost impossible to break. Having an ill adult child is not rare.

For Annette, her relationship with Justin, Sophia's husband, was important to maintaining her connection with her daughter. "Justin and I worked really well together. I feel like I am a little different than some, but again it depends on the age of your child and how you always got along." The adult child's degree of independence, other adult relationships, and relationship with parents will put the parents more or less in the shadows. It is variable and individual. Sophia seemed to look to Annette first for decisions that involved her medical care and then to Justin. For questions about married life and social decisions, she looked to Justin first. It seemed to be a functional and equitable division for everyone.

The ability to work many different things out, particularly related to Sophia's illness, greatly affected each of their experiences. Annette was realistic. "I do not think I was in the shadows as much as some parents are. I think that a lot of times they are in the shadows because of previous incidents with the partner. For example, if there were issues between Justin and me, because of his legal status as the husband, I would be pushed into the shadows. As her husband, he was the legal decision maker. I do think those previous relationships are key."

These decisions included how to best meet her physical needs. They worked together, with Sophia's input, to control pain, manage side effects of the medication, and increase her physical activity. While Sophia was in the hospital, Annette and Justin took turns staying overnight with her. They got to know the care staff well. Annette would bring back stories about the hospital unit "gossip."

It was also a joint decision to call in hospice for end-of-life care. This difficult decision made it possible to care for Sophia at home and keep her comfortable. Her care needs included a hospital bed for ease of movement and care, medications to relieve pain and trouble breathing, ice chips when she couldn't eat but complained of a dry mouth, and hand and foot rubs with her favorite lotion. Physical needs are so important.

# Conclusion

Some of the skills necessary to care for your seriously ill adult child will be caring for their physical needs. Remember how absolutely essential that was when they were newborns and then growing through the toddler, school age, and teen years. It is no less important now. The needs of the seriously ill include the need to breathe easily, the need for food and water, the need to be free from pain, and the need to overcome fatigue. There are others, and the "By the Way..." section will give you additional resources.

# References

Bernardin, J.C. (1997). *The gift of peace.* Chicago, IL: Loyola Press.

Mann, F., & Carr, E. (2006). *Pain management.* Oxford, UK: Blackwell Publishing.

National Comprehensive Cancer Network. (2011). *NCCN Clinical Practice Guidelines in Oncology: Cancer-related fatigue* [v.1.2012]. Retrieved from http://www.nccn.org/professionals/physician_gls/pdf/fatigue.pdf

Wanchai, A., Armer, J.M., & Stewart, B.R. (2011). Nonpharmacologic supportive strategies to promote quality of life in patients experiencing cancer-related fatigue: A systematic review. *Clinical Journal of Oncology Nursing,* *15,* 203–214. doi:10.1188/11.CJON.203-214

**By the Way...**

- Healthcare professionals, especially palliative care experts, know a lot about managing physical symptoms. *Palliative care* is supportive care that includes the management of physical, psychological, and spiritual suffering anywhere throughout the illness continuum. A palliative care consultation may be requested. Do not be afraid of this or assume it means hospice or end-of-life care. Palliative care specialists are experts at controlling a large variety of physical symptoms.

- Caring for physical needs of an adult often means taking care of or helping them with activities of daily living. These include personal care such as bathing, dressing, toileting, and feeding; transportation; maintaining a household by cooking, cleaning, laundering, and grocery shopping; and clerical tasks such as banking, paying bills, and making appointments.

- Recognize that a commitment to care for someone requires energy and strength, not just the heart or willingness. Care for yourself as well (see Chapter 8. What About Me? Caring for Yourself).

- If opioids (also sometimes known as narcotics) are prescribed to relieve symptoms of pain or breathlessness, do not object. They are excellent drugs for these problems, and when managed by a professional, they will not lead to addiction.

- Some good online resources for caregivers include the National Cancer Institute (www.cancer.gov), Rosalynn Carter Institute for Caregiving (www.rosalynncarter.org), Endo Pharmaceuticals (www.painaction.com), Caregiver Resource Network (www.caregiverresource.net), Family Caregiver Alliance (http://caregiver.org), National Caregivers Library (www.caregiverslibrary.org), and Today's Caregiver (http://caregiver.com).

- Sometimes healthcare agencies offer classes in caregiving. Generally they are free or have a minimal cost. Check in your area for this possibility.

- Online fertility resources include American Society for Reproductive Medicine (www.asrm.org), American Fertility Association (www.theafa.org), and Fertile Hope (www.fertilehope.org).

# CHAPTER 4

# THE ROLLER COASTER:
# Emotional Care

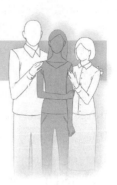

*You don't really understand human nature unless you know why a child on a merry-go-round will wave at his parent every time around and why his parent will always wave back.*

—William D. Tammeus

## Patti Beach's Story

As a freshman at Ohio State University (OSU), Kim called just about every day, usually as she walked across campus, and the timing of that call in early January was not unusual in any way.

"I've been bleeding."

"What do you mean?"

"With my poop, I have blood."

"Kimmie, everything that is red is not blood," as a nurse, I automatically replied.

But it was blood and it continued. First diagnosed as hemorrhoids, the bleeding continued. As the snow turned to slush, the bleeding continued, not worse but no better. Our family doctor instructed us to see a specialist. It would be quite a while before she could get an appointment. This wait was made even longer because Kim did not want to disrupt her schooling and her schedule was pretty tight. So, one delay led to another. She felt the same, no complaints except bleeding with her stools. In fact, she even went to Florida with friends for spring break and had a great time.

Four months later on a Sunday night in April, Kim called crying. She confessed that her bleeding had increased; she was not having any normal stools, only diarrhea. Her bowel movements were frequent with several throughout the night. She was tired, sometimes light-headed, and felt she couldn't keep up with her studies.

When I called the family doctor to try to expedite the appointment with the specialist, he seemed upset and uncharacteristically almost rude. Although Kim was legally an adult, she still looked to me for all direction regarding medical care and health problems. I thought maybe we were being difficult but Kim was getting so much sicker. Now I wonder if it was difficult for him because Kim was 19 and he wanted to treat her as an adult patient. Maybe he didn't know what my role in this illness was. This made it harder to ask questions and ask for help.

In May, Kim saw the specialist, a high-energy woman, quick with a presumptive diagnosis of ulcerative colitis. She did not sit down to talk to us but quickly came in and out of the exam room. A colonoscopy confirmed the diagnosis of ulcerative colitis. Medications were prescribed, diet modifications were recommended, and assurances were made that this would "take care of everything." But the bleeding continued, and Kim was hospitalized to receive three units of blood.

It was during this hospitalization that the family doctor saw her for the first time since the initial office visit about three or four months earlier. His conversation angered me. I was a bystander, at best. He started with what a difficult diagnosis ulcerative colitis was and when he had seen other cases he wondered, that if faced with it himself, would he just choose to have his colon removed in the beginning?

I thought, "What?! Who needed surgery? Who was facing a colostomy to make life better? Surely not my beautiful 19-year-old daughter!"

I made many calls during this hospitalization to notify family and close friends about what was happening. Visitors, cards, calls, and flowers all helped. Some of those who were there for us were a surprise . . . and only a few melted away, never to be heard from during this time.

It was also during this three-day hospitalization that I started what would become my pattern. When my husband, Kim's dad, was visiting, I would leave the hospital to shower and clean up, returning always to spend the night. Her care was very good but I could not trust her to be alone with only staff. She was so young and would hesitate to speak up if she needed something. She wouldn't want to bother anyone.

Staying the night also gave me some insight into how little she was sleeping. Because she was living at the university, I only had her reports of "I'm getting up a lot." Indeed, she was getting up almost every hour with bleeding and mucous diarrhea. She had a lot of abdominal pain, especially after eating. Ulcerative colitis's hallmarks seem to be bloody stools that are accompanied by abdominal pain and cramping, "dry heaves of the rectum."

After the blood transfusions and medication changes, Kim returned to school. She was only getting up two or three times a night. Her bowel movements were still mostly diarrhea with blood, but there was a rare one without visible blood. We were hopeful.

Frequent phone calls, made easily with cell phones, were important but sometimes difficult. Kim kept me informed, allowing me to offer support. But it is hard to be reminded that your child is ill, that she is hurting. Sometimes I hated to answer the phone; I knew it might ruin my day. Even with the separation of distance, your day goes as your child's does.

In June, Kim saw another gastroenterologist specialist. He was a good clinician, very kind, and skillfully negotiated between patient and mother. More medications were prescribed.

The summer had been blessedly quiet. Kim went back to OSU to begin her sophomore year in September, hopeful that she would stay well. About halfway through the quarter she noticed blood in her stool, although not every day, not every time. Some of her stools were still normal, without diarrhea. I thought, "Nothing to worry about." Then I thought, "Better to have the doctor tell us it was nothing to worry about." Kim reluctantly agreed to let me call him. Any amount of denial did not serve us well with ulcerative colitis.

The doctor said that Kim was no longer in remission. Her remission had lasted about two or three months. Again, more medications were prescribed, including nightly enemas. We, and the physician, were confident of remission by Thanksgiving, three weeks away. Good days and bad nights continued.

So, how does a college coed handle giving herself nightly enemas? She does her best! For Kim, her friends and roommates were great support. They were curious but also empathetic. She was not left on her own. I think because she was open about what she was going through, she connected with several others on campus who were suffering with inflammatory bowel disease, either ulcerative colitis or Crohn disease. Even with the support and positive hopeful attitude, the physical disease raged on. Attitude is important, but it is not everything.

Kim seemed to handle just about all of this with flexibility and some humor. She tried hard to continue with school and social activities. During this time she met a young man who understood because his brother also had ulcerative colitis. By December, the bleeding stopped and her stools were more formed, or as she described them, "fluffy." We were hopeful again.

June, 18 months since the bleeding started, the ulcerative colitis came back in full force. All Kim's bowel movements were with blood or blood alone. We scrutinized the medications. We scrutinized the diet. We scrutinized the supplements. What were we missing?

Was there someone somewhere else who could help? Try something we have not? I made three different appointments with GI specialists at a world-renowned medical center about two hours from our home thinking, "I will take whichever doctor I can get in with first." Of course, these multiple appointments screwed up the computer, and we got kicked out of all appointments except the last one. Not what I wanted.

That November, finally, the long-awaited visit to the specialist had arrived. We met with an inflammatory bowel specialist, a thoughtful man and according to Kim, "the smartest doctor I ever had." We spent two hours with him, reviewing her history and discussing options.

Then before I knew it, we were discussing removing the colon. He turned to me and asked what I thought. "You keep your body parts as long as you can," I answered with some déjà vu back to the family doctor's conversation during Kim's first hospitalization.

"True," he replied, "as long as they're working."

"Now your daughter has no quality of life," he went on. "She is not sleeping at night, is always tired and relying on blood transfusions. Is this how she should continue to live? The surgeons will tell you that removing the colon is a cure. It is not. But she will feel better."

We met for 30 minutes with a colorectal surgeon. He did promise a cure. He would remove the colon, also called the large intestine, and rectum, fashion an internal J-pouch to hold stool from the end of the small intestine, also called the ileum, and then attach the ileum to the anus. So, for a few months, she would have an ileostomy, a bag on her abdomen that would drain stool. This would require two surgeries, the first to remove the colon, make the J-pouch, and attach the ileum to the anus. This pouch would not function for three months, until all was healed. During that time, stool would be diverted to the ileostomy bag. After all the surgeries, Kim would have four to seven oatmeal-like bowel movements a day without urgency or bleeding. Her bowel movements would be the "normal" way, not through a bag on her abdomen.

Kim's expectations for this visit were not very high and mine were hopeful of a miracle drug; it is fair to say we both left there surprised. Seemingly overnight I went from fighting surgery to accepting it. Surgery was scheduled for three weeks, over Christmas break.

In the meantime, a physician friend suggested acupuncture. When I told my husband about this, I thought he was going to do acupuncture on me right there in the kitchen! But he is a wise man and he walked away, letting me investigate this option. After talking to the acupuncturist, it was clear this was not an option. She was honest; she had no experience with ulcerative colitis, and Kim was too sick. Later when I told Kim that she could be confident that she tried or looked into all options, she said, "No, I'm OK but you can be sure, mom." She was right.

Having a seriously ill child, no matter the age of the child, is difficult. The age and developmental stage, particularly the degree of independence, will greatly influence the parent and child's responses. This chapter will sort out some of the emotional responses and give suggestions for how a parent can best help.

When an adult child is seriously ill, the parent often feels invisible. It is probably not the first time. Being introduced as someone's parent, rather than an individual with a name, is common. Invisibility occurs in other circumstances as well. Although parents are neither invisible nor the center of this illness drama, they do have feelings.

## Emotions

Emotions: everyone has them. They are feelings; mental states that are subjective and not experienced as a conscious thought. Physiologic changes accompany emotions that may or may not be apparent to oneself or to others.

Emotions are what the person experiencing them says they are. Everyone can name them but not control them. This is important to remember, particularly when experiencing negative emotions. What can be controlled is how one responds to them, but not whether they happen.

As mentioned in Chapter 1, something that may not often be talked about is that you can have negative emotions toward loved ones, including your children. This is normal. These emotions might be anger, sadness, disappointment, anxiety, depression, or others. They are normal, acceptable, and do not lessen your love for your child.

Accepting any negative emotions you may experience toward your child is even more difficult when your child is sick. You love your child and have cared for him for many years. But you can still have negative feelings. However, it may be this investment of years of care and caring that leads parents to want to deal with any ambivalence or tension created by the tug and pull of positive and negative emotions constructively rather than destructively.

Marilee and Joseph felt this tension and ambivalence. It was almost palpable when their 33-year-old daughter, Jeannine, had been receiving dialysis for the past two years because of kidney failure caused by a congenital condition and was on the national transplant list. They had been there for her, helped provide transportation and frequently babysat her two children. When she was tired or depressed, they continued to help, often biting back hurtful words. Now, recently retired, they were planning a cross-country driving trip with several friends. Their long-held dream was to visit several national parks and monuments. They were excited; the trip would be crowned with a visit to Yosemite National Park. Along with the planning, they must also account for Jeannine. How should they handle their commitments to her? She said they should go on the trip. What if an emergency arose while they were gone? Could they be reached and get back home in time to help? Particularly they were concerned that if a donor kidney became available they would want to be with her. Should they give up the trip? They seemed too old to have to still be worrying about their children. What if they did not get another opportunity to travel this road? Finally, they decided to go on the trip, check in with Jeannine at regular intervals, and always let her know how they could be reached.

When someone in the family has a serious illness, many difficult decisions must be made. People make the best decisions they can with the information and circumstances they are given. As one mother said, "Nobody chooses to make a bad decision, but you can't make decisions based on how your child might react, or at least it is not the only thing to consider." Many parents enjoyed raising their children and also enjoyed the freedom that returned when their children left home to live independently. However, in most cases, parents still want to help.

This help will be offered no matter the age of the child. How can a parent offer help that will be accepted but not stifling? How to be constructive? Adult children consistently say, "Treat us like adults." They want advice when they ask for it. Unsolicited advice is rarely taken well and will increase tensions. In addition, advice should be given kindly. If it is meant to help, it should be given in a spirit of helpfulness. Angry, critical words will harm a relationship, no matter the age of the parent or child.

Parents can ask what help is needed. If it is running errands, babysitting, or walking the dog, do what you can. When you can't help, offer an alternative if one is available.

Finally, after you have done what you can and offered any words of wisdom you have, *stop*. Your child gets to decide what to accept or decline. Accept his decision, and do not nag. Do not begrudge him if your advice is not taken. Remember, it is not about you. This is not always easy because you tend to think that you, as the parent, know what is best. Work at accepting your child's decisions. This will not eliminate the ambivalence but improves the chances of constructive resolution.

## Worry and Hope

Worry describes those negative and intrusive thoughts about the possible future. No one worries about the past. As many have asked, "When do parents stop worrying about their children?" "Can it be that parents are sentenced to a lifetime of worry?" It is the progression of changing worries as your child grows—about stitches, grades, returning home safely in the early morning hours—that is never ending. Perhaps anything that occurs unexpectedly leads to worry. Certainly a sick child leads to worry.

The popular press and academic literature may lead you to believe that parents only worry about young children. That is not true. Parents worry about their children no matter their age. Many have said, "When your kids are young, your worries are small; when they grow up, you worry about bigger things." Perhaps these worries seem bigger because they are less under your control. When your child is small, to keep her safe, you hold her hand as she crosses the street. It is a more difficult question about how to keep a child safe who is walking alone across campus on a dark night. Parents trust that their child will be watchful, maybe carry a can of mace in her backpack. When your child suffers with a serious illness, the worries change and are more serious. It is not because of the age of the child but because of the loss of control, the helplessness.

Information helps decrease worry. Decreasing your own worrying and anxiousness can have positive effects on your child's adjustment, too. The information you seek may be personal to your child and about the illness. Although the need for health information is great, the sharing of personal information is not free. It comes with personal and legal restrictions.

When parents are interacting with healthcare professionals, they must be aware of the legalities. It is the adult child's responsibility to decide who receives which details about his illness. Legally, parents have no recognized rights to information if their child is 18 years of age or older. At this age, healthcare law gives people the right to make their own decisions. Confidentiality must be maintained at all times and healthcare professionals are extremely aware of this. This includes the diagnosis and all aspects of treatment. That is in compliance with the Health Insurance Portability and Accountability Act (HIPAA) and is discussed in more detail in Chapter 9.

Information about the illness can be found in written, verbal, or online formats. No matter what form the information takes, always consider how credible it is. Some questions to ask:

• What is the source of the information?
• How do you know this information is true?
• Is it pertinent to your circumstances?

Talking to others also lessens worrying. You can learn a lot when you talk to others, especially that you are not alone. You may learn something very helpful or totally useless, but you are now less alone. For example, acupuncture was not a viable option for Kim. But I had to check that out to know that I had not overlooked any possibilities. After that I also knew, again, that both my husband and my friend were right there going through this illness with Kim and me.

Hope and worry are two sides of the same coin. Hope changes, but it is rare that it is completely absent. It is natural to want a cure, but this is not always possible. So perhaps hope changes to control of disease or for a graduation or to attend a wedding celebration. Realistic hope is the belief that you can improve a situation and feel happiness. Hope is an ongoing choice. There are many sources of hope, both internal and external. It is important to define your hope and share it with your child.

One source of hope is the belief in the treatment plan. Often the loss of control contributes to many of the negative feelings associated with a serious illness. Belief in the treatment plan, a clear plan of action, even if it is not under your control or if it changes, is important for coping. A clear plan, implemented in a predictable and effective manner, is part of hopefulness.

# Independence and Dependence

The emotion a parent may feel in response to an adult child's illness is in part related to the child's developmental stage. "Adult" encompasses years and decades. Anne Grinyer, a medical sociologist in England, has looked at young adults with cancer and the effect that the illness has on life trajectories and biographies. For the young adult, cancer affects their education, careers, life plans, friendships, appearance, sexuality and fertility, future earnings, and independence. Independence at this developmental stage is still fragile. Many younger adults are either still living at home with their parents or have just left home for education or jobs. Her research suggests an age-appropriate approach for both the parent and the healthcare professional (personal communication, August 20, 2010).

The young adult's loss of independence during medical treatment may be seen very differently by the young adult than the parent. The parent may see it as the price that must be paid for good care and treatment. The young adult child may see it as a much larger forfeiture. They may long for the "normal" that they see with their friends and peers.

The issue of perspective with a serious illness strikingly shows the difference between young adults and their parents. Parents tend to be very interested in the outcome, whereas the young adult values the experience more. The young adult child is more process-driven and heavily weighs the quality of life throughout the treatment experience. For example, Grinyer (2009) found that parents focus on the cure but the young adults pay more attention to how they are treated; aspects of care such as privacy and open visiting hours for friends are very important (Grinyer, 2009).

Grinyer tells of a young Australian man who was ill with leukemia. Despite this illness, he wanted to travel with his friends to England, stopping in other countries along the route. His parents let him go and were never to see him alive again. His disease relapsed with a vengeance while he was on holiday. He died in England before they were able to reach his bedside. In an understated summation Grinyer says, "It is incredibly hard for parents to see their child predecease them." The parents of this young man are not bitter. They were supporting their child in doing what he felt compelled to do with as little interference from the disease as possible (personal communication, August 20, 2010).

For an adult child who is older and had established living independently from the parents before the illness struck, the scenarios around illness and treatment are often different. The child may live near the parents or a distance from them. This distance may be more than geographic. The older ill adult child often has a job and family of his own. His responsibilities and day-to-day attention may lie elsewhere than with the parent. This may be what leads some to categorize parents of adult children as "extended family." Very few parents feel like they are extended family, no matter the age of the child. When the child is sick, the impulse to parent, to be near and help, seems to be even stronger.

That doesn't mean that ambivalence disappears. Sylvia reported feeling conflicted about how her 47-year-old daughter was caring for herself after a diagnosis of sarcoidosis, an inflammatory disease that was attacking her lungs. Sylvia thought she should seek care with a specialist but her daughter disagreed. "When she was a baby, I took good care of her. She was born premature and needed specialist care and we did that. Why can't she do the same for herself now?"

Sometimes the life cycle of dependence and independence does a full rotation and the elderly parent becomes dependent on the adult child. Social worker Amanda Sager, whose clients are elderly, sees worry toward their ill children even in those parents who live in an assisted living or extended care facility. Living in an institutional setting has already isolated these parents from many familiar routines. They rely on the adult child to visit and keep them in touch. This may include providing their favorite foods, bringing grandchildren to visit, or doing some laundry. If the adult child becomes seriously ill and the visiting decreases, it may further isolate the parent. Mixed emotions are common. These negative feelings need to be recognized, acknowledged, and accepted. After that, there are ways to foster staying connected. Sager believes that connection is the cornerstone of adjusting to changes. She suggests allowing the elderly parent to accompany their adult child during physician visits and be given frequent information updates either by telephone or in person. Information is often the key to emotional adjustment (personal communication, August 5, 2010).

Sager has often counseled residents when they are angry at their child or feel guilty because they can't help their child. "Residents are ashamed of these negative feelings. I help them see that these feelings are understandable and that these are difficult situations," she explained. "Parents need to know that changes are going to happen; they will adjust; their family will survive" (personal communication, August 5, 2010). The support and information they receive from family, friends, and caregivers is key to their recovery and survival.

# Grief

Grief is the price we pay for love. It is "a person's emotional response to the event of loss" (Corless, 2006, p. 532). Although the term *grief* is frequently associated with dying, it is not just a response to death but to any important loss. It may be about the loss of independence or health or status or future dreams. It may be in response to changes that have occurred or will occur.

Dr. Elisabeth Kübler-Ross's work with grief in the 1960s and 1970s is well known and often quoted. She was a pioneer in explaining grief and the final chapter of living. *On Death and Dying,* her classic work, describes the stages of grief as denial, anger, bargaining, depression, and acceptance (Kübler-Ross, 1969). Today, we understand these better not as stages through which everyone progresses in an orderly fashion but as tasks and possible responses to grief. An individual may or may not experience some or all of these.

As it turns out, most people may be born to cope with emotional adversity. George Bonanno, emotions expert and authority on bereavement at Columbia University's Teachers College, contends that we are hardwired to deal with losses and that grief can actually deepen interpersonal connections (Bonanno, 2009). Often, new meanings are discerned at the most difficult of times and through tragedy.

Susan and Gary had two children, a boy and a girl. Both children had been star athletes in high school, popular, well-liked, and average scholars. Steven, their oldest, developed substance abuse problems in college. Alcohol, narcotics, and cocaine were all part of his painful addictions. Several rehabilitation efforts failed. He came home to live; they kicked him out; he returned; again he began abusing drugs and alcohol; he left without a word. Run-ins with the law further strained their relationship. On his 30th birthday, they did not know how to contact him. By this time, Susan and Gary didn't know his phone number or address. But then, the next year, he called. Could he come home? He had nowhere else to go. He was ill. The previous years had seen accumulating and multiple infections and now he had end-stage liver disease. Could he come home? "Yes," they said, "the door is open again."

Can illness heal the hurt? Bonanno's work and observations through the years give a positive answer. Yes, it is never too late to try to return to a relationship that may have been damaged. The strength of the parent-child attachment can survive damage and hurts. Someone must be willing to make the first move, and often it is the parent who must make the initial gesture toward reconciliation. Making the first move is risky and may be met with rejection. It is important for the parent to be constructive and willing to see the child's point of view and to work through the hurt. These efforts can result in reconciliation and a better understanding of your child as an adult. Emotions are positive and negative and are part of the fabric of our lives.

## Patti's Story

In December, almost two years since the bleeding started, the day of Kim's surgery to remove her colon arrived. After she was taken back to prepare for surgery, we noticed the monitors with updates on patient status. Despite the monitor updates, we were called to speak with the surgeon about three hours after the procedure started or about halfway through the expected surgical time. This early meeting could not be good news—and it wasn't.

Kim did well through the surgery, we were told, the colon was removed but the tissues were too fragile to form the internal J-pouch. The surgeon would have to take her back to surgery in about six months and make the J-pouch and then again three months later to close the ileostomy. So, three surgeries instead of two; nine months with an ileostomy instead of three; one more medical plan that did not go as planned. The goal remained the same, a cure. It would just take longer. In a year, the results would be the same. The struggle continued, but still we had a plan. That was important even when the plan kept changing. Being able to give voice to what is next gave us hope and confidence. It felt as though we knew what was happening. Was it real or a façade? We didn't really look at that question too closely, probably because of the fragility of our plan.

I formed my own little virtual support network with e-mails. About 30 family and friends got regular updates, and I eagerly read their replies. It kept me in touch with our real lives, lives that did not include the hospital. Prayers also helped.

Kim's boyfriend was a big support. He visited regularly and handled all the medical paraphernalia well. Once I handed him all the postoperative tubes as we were helping Kim out of bed to go for a walk. She said, "Don't have him hold that. It's gross."

I looked at him and he replied, "It's OK. I couldn't do it except for Kim." All the parenting in the world can't replace that kind of acceptance.

Eleven days after surgery, we were sent home. Finally, we were home. Christmas came, and I was glad Dan insisted we decorate as always before the surgery. It was good to be home.

Family and friends continued to surround us literally and figuratively. I believe the best healing occurs in your own environment. Kim's boyfriend continued to act like all of his girlfriends had had ileostomies. That was a blessing, too.

Kim was always independent caring for her ileostomy. I know she didn't like it, but she did what she had to do. Of course, I bought her any clothes she thought helped her look better. This generosity was sorely tested on one shopping trip when I questioned whether she really needed a new, quite expensive, purse.

"Mom, I don't have a colon!"

"Everyone has one and they are very overrated," I assured her. Humor helps. No purse.

Colon-less Kim returned to OSU spring quarter. Spring became summer. She found a bathing suit that flattered her thin figure with the ileostomy and the right supplies to put over it for swimming. Surgeries were scheduled for the end of May and August.

In August, nine months after her first surgery, Kim's ileostomy was closed, almost a nonevent. She came home after an overnight stay.

Now more than three years since Kim had her colon removed and more than five years since she started bleeding, she is doing well but still struggles with sleeping all night whether because of habit or frequent bowel movements. She eats well and what she likes. Annual follow-ups are the routine, but she will still have intermittent bouts of frequent diarrhea sometimes related to an infection called pouchitis. She is definitely better colon-less.

## Conclusion

Worry is something every parent knows and so is hope, especially when your child is seriously ill. Hope may change depending on the circumstances, but it never disappears completely. As you go through these difficulties, positive and negative emotions are expected, and both may even sometimes be directed at your child. Although the emotions are not under your control, your actions are. Constructive actions may include seeking information, having a plan, and maintaining normalcy. Offering your child these, with hope, will help in a tough situation.

## References

Bonanno, G. (2009). *The other side of sadness.* New York, NY: Basic Books.

Corless, I. (2006). Bereavement. In B. Ferrell & N. Coyle (Eds.), *Textbook of palliative nursing* (2nd ed., pp. 531–544). New York, NY: Oxford University Press.

Grinyer, A. (2009). Contrasting parental perspectives with those of teenagers and young adults with cancer: Comparing the findings from two qualitative studies. *European Journal of Oncology Nursing, 13,* 200–206.

Kübler-Ross, E. (1969). *On death and dying.* New York, NY: Macmillan.

## By the Way...

- Remember that your child is an adult.
- You cannot control your emotions or feelings, only your actions.
- Positive actions to help your child include obtaining information, maintaining normalcy, accommodating the child's wishes, working together, and understanding your child's point of view.
- Carefully balance routine and flexibility.
- Keep a journal for your thoughts, dates, numbers and names, inspirational quotes, maybe even a joke or cartoon that makes you laugh. It is helpful to keep all this important information in one place and to choose a journal that is attractive to you so that you are more likely to use it.
- Talk to others for support, advice, and information. You will never know what others know or have been through if you don't talk about what you are going through.
- Web-based support is a growing area and should be explored. Many hospitals provide a Web-based blog where you can give out information that you want others to have and they can respond to you. This support, especially from a distance, can prove invaluable. Examples include My Care Community (www.MyCare Community.org) and CaringBridge (www.caringbridge.org).
- Staying the night may be important depending on the age and independence level of your child. No matter the age, frequent visiting is a way to stay in touch, offer support, and identify ways to help.
- Cards, telephone calls, flowers, and gifts are all ways to stay in touch and show support.
- If you cannot be with your child, devise a convenient system to share information. It might be with phone calls, texting, or e-mails. If your child gives permission for you to talk with healthcare providers, communicate this with them and understand their process and protocols. There may be passwords involved.
- Know your care providers by name. The nurse is often an especially good source of information and help.
- Have someone who will let you cry. This doesn't have to be the person you are closest to and in fact, that may not work well.
- When asked, give advice gently.

# CHAPTER 5

# EVERYTHING HAS A PRICE TAG:
# Financial Care

*Making the decision to have a child—it's momentous.*
*It is to decide forever to have your heart go walking*
*around outside your body.*

– Elizabeth Stone

## Connie's Story

Mark was 26 years old and a promising business entrepreneur. Three years out of college with a business degree, he was living in a large city 200 miles from home and well on his way to financial success as a business consultant. Ironically, Mark did not take some of his own business advice: prepare for the unexpected. Like many young adults, he found health insurance coverage too expensive and "not really needed." He was too old to be covered under his parents' health insurance policy. Besides, he couldn't remember the last time he was sick enough to see a doctor. His mother is a nurse and, although she worried that he didn't have health insurance, she did not think it was so essential that she should pay for it herself. Mark would "take care of that later." On a weekend trip home, Mark showed his mother a lump under the skin in his chest. An x-ray and subsequent biopsy diagnosed the tumor as treatable lymphoma, a cancer of the white blood cells. Mark was rich in dreams and had little more to pay the staggering cost of cancer treatment.

Finances are hard to talk about. In fact, it falls in the top three along with politics and religion as the most emotionally charged topics for people to talk about. Illness, however, is expensive. Predicting the cost of any given test, medicine, procedure, or therapy is simply a gamble. Costs vary depending on where you live, where you seek care, even whether you have health insurance or are paying out of your own pocket. Even more difficult to predict are the indirect costs of illness such as lost wages, expenses incurred to travel for treatment, child care, and food. When talking about serious illness, it is necessary to talk about money.

The purpose of this chapter is to recognize the financial burden that illness may place on an individual and a family. This is not a debate about our healthcare system or a soliloquy on what changes are needed. Rather, the chapter is an introduction into the common financial hurdles encountered when serious illness occurs and how parents of seriously ill adult children can help without compromising their own financial well-being.

It often feels wrong or uncaring to inquire about the cost of medical care. "There is no price too high for good health care," is a frequently heard phrase. Yet, insurance companies, hospitals, physicians, pharmacies, and therapists do not allow us to choose any healthcare treatment we want. Healthcare decisions are made every day based on cost. Insurance companies decide what they will or will not pay for and patients decide whether the co-pay or the length and side effects of treatment are worth the money. The strain and stress of financial worries can add to the concerns about disease treatment.

Parents want to help in any way possible. "I would have sold everything I had to make her well and keep her family intact," said Addie. Addie and her husband sold their retirement home in Florida and he returned to work at age 70 to help their daughter following a diagnosis of multiple sclerosis.

"I found myself buying clothes that would fit over my daughter's colostomy in every color in her size," said Susan.

"I decided that I could just work a few more years. Then my son's family could live with me, and I could afford the extra costs in food and utilities," said Katerina.

But, what is best for parents and ill adult children? What is a reasonable financial commitment for parents? How can parents make the best decisions for their situation in life?

## First, Whoa! Slow Down

Almost no financial decision needs to be made overnight, advises Nolan Baker (personal communication, March 13, 2012), investment professional and cofounder of The Retirement Guys (www.retirementguysnetwork.com) in Maumee, Ohio. Do your homework. What is really needed? "Have the tough talk with your adult children," Baker recommends. Listen carefully to what they say they need. Work together to make sure that your help is long lasting. Although giving money is an obvious choice, often it will not help the most. Consider helping by using your world experience. In other words, offer practical help and knowledge of available resources.

# Give Knowledge

"Knowledge is power," said Sir Francis Bacon. Learn about resources that will provide money and services to pay for direct and indirect costs of health care. You can be an invaluable asset to your adult child if you obtain needed information about healthcare financing and ways to negotiate the best prices and services. When you become a powerhouse of knowledge, you can help your adult child save thousands of dollars in healthcare costs and access useful resources.

Remember that if you don't have written permission to speak on behalf of your child, you will not be able to get any health information or discuss finances with healthcare providers. The Health Insurance Portability and Accountability Act (HIPAA) of 1996 provides privacy protection for healthcare information and allows adults to name persons who may speak on their behalf when they are unable to do so.

Mark Clair, an Ohio attorney (personal communication, March 13, 2012), strongly recommends that your adult child complete two pertinent documents: A healthcare power of attorney (HC-POA) and an authorization to release personal health information. The HC-POA allows adults to name one person to make healthcare decisions on his or her behalf *only when he or she is incapacitated and not able to make those decisions.* That person is referred to as the "surrogate" or "proxy" decision maker. The authorization to release personal health information allows a person (in this case, your adult child) to give consent or permission for one or more individuals to receive information about that person's health care and insurance. Although the HC-POA usually names just one person, more than one person may be given permission to receive health information. This permission is required to receive any information at all, including progress during hospitalization, insurance coverage, or qualifications required for additional services. Most organizations require written consent. Your state may have preferred documents, especially for the HC-POA.

**Patient Consent to Share Information Form Example**

I consent to share my health information with _____
*(fill in the blank here with the name of your adult child's doctor or hospital)*

I, _____, *(your adult child's name goes here)* give permission to allow _____ *(put your name here)* to share _____ *(fill in the blank here with everything that your adult child is giving permission for you to see, such as "all my insurance, billing, and medical information")* with the following exceptions _____. *(if there are things your adult child does not want you to see, put that in this blank)*

Signed name of patient *(your adult child's name goes here)*

_____

Date of birth_____ *(your adult child's date of birth goes here to help the physician or organization verify they are releasing the correct person's information)*

Printed name of patient *(your adult child's printed name goes here)*

_____

Date_____

Notary Public seal and signature_____

This consent is valid until _____or one year from the date above.

# Insurance

Understanding health insurance policies can be a challenge. When reading an insurance policy there are specific questions to think about and for your adult child to understand. With your child's permission, you can save your child time and money by finding answers to health insurance-related questions.

---

### Questions to Ask About Your Child's Healthcare Insurance Coverage

What services are covered that may be needed for your adult child's medical care?

Are doctor's office visits, mental health services, and physical therapy covered?

Is hospice a benefit? What about home care?

Is there a cap or limit on how long the services may be provided or how much the insurance company will pay for the duration of the policy?

Is it necessary to see certain physicians or healthcare organizations in order for the insurance company to pay the most?

If you go to a provider that the insurance company does not approve, can they refuse to pay?

What are the co-pays, or the amount of money that the patient must pay in addition to the amount the insurance company pays?

What is the deductible, or the amount that must be paid out of pocket before the insurance company begins to pay? Is the deductible amount the cost for the whole family or for each individual in the family?

What if your adult child needs a physician, treatment, or medicine that is not covered? Can the insurance company really refuse to pay for something your adult child's doctor recommends? (Yes.)

Is there anything that can be done? (Yes again.)

---

Health insurance companies are acutely aware of how complex and costly health care is. It is both compassionate and fiscally prudent of health insurance companies to provide patients with as much information as possible to manage their diseases and the cost of healthcare services. Health insurance companies employ physicians to identify medical standards of care and best medical practices so that patients can receive the most up-to-date, safe care.

Coordination of medical care and support services is very important when complex illness occurs. This coordination may be provided by insurance case managers. A case manager is often a registered nurse with experience caring for people who are ill as well as knowledge of the healthcare system and healthcare financing. When adult patients have illnesses that are very complicated and costly, a case manager is often assigned to oversee the healthcare services used and the patient's response to treatment. Case managers are often the most connected contacts in an insurance company. In other words, if they don't know an answer, they may well know whom to speak with to get the best answer. If you have questions about health insurance, call and ask to speak to a case manager.

## No Health Insurance

When your adult child doesn't have health insurance or can't afford co-pays and deductibles, negotiation may be key. Many people erroneously believe that healthcare fees are the same from any given hospital, physician's office, laboratory, or rehabilitation facility. That is definitely not true. The fact is that insurance companies negotiate a price for everything they agree to pay for: hospital care, diagnostic services, medications, therapies, and physician services. Those negotiated prices are usually much lower than the prices charged for people who are directly paying their own bills. How much different can those costs be? The Agency for Healthcare Research and Quality (AHRQ, 2009) publishes statistics on hospital-based care in the United States. Its latest report showed that the average charges per hospital stay were $30,700. With an average hospital stay of 4.6 days, this cost is $6,674/day. Compare those charges with the costs paid by insurance companies. For the same hospital stay, the average amount insurance companies paid was $9,200 or $2,000/day (AHRQ, 2009). This is more than a threefold difference between what those with health insurance paid for services and the amount paid by those who pay privately or "out of pocket."

Even for those with private insurance, co-pays and deductibles can vary between as high as $5,950 for an individual and $11,900 for a family policy. A deductible is the amount of money that must be paid first before the health insurance company begins to pay. Co-pay is a set amount of money you pay in addition to what the insurance company pays for the service.

Hospitals and other healthcare providers are often open to negotiating payment plans or discounts. If you are paying out of pocket, do not hesitate to ask for a charge that is similar to that paid by insurance companies. Make an appointment to talk with the billing office to discuss options. An important note: negotiating prices for healthcare services is best done before those services are given. Trying to negotiate a lower price after services are rendered may not be as straightforward.

Consider negotiating a payment plan with an end date. For example, a payment plan of $200/month for five years may be less than billed, but enough to satisfy the healthcare provider. A word of caution: missed payments may nullify the contract, so be careful that you can afford what you agree to in a payment plan.

It is not necessary to have health insurance provided by an employer for it to be affordable. Many large insurance companies are competing for the non-employer market. The choices are many and prices are often competitive. Ask the public librarian for assistance if you are unsure about searching the Internet for "insurance for one" or "individual and family health insurance."

If your ill adult child is recently unemployed and worked for a company with 20 or more employees, he or she may qualify for the Consolidated Omnibus Budget Reconciliation Act (COBRA) (U.S. Department of Labor, n.d.). COBRA permits extension of employer health benefit provisions. This program allows individuals to purchase the same health insurance as offered to other company employees. The full cost of the premium must be paid by the person and may or may not be more affordable than independently purchasing individual or family coverage. Other important restrictions apply with COBRA. Ask the company's benefits department for more information.

Your adult child may qualify for public insurance, such as Medicaid or Medicare. These state and federally funded programs provide comprehensive health care and serve people who meet certain income, age, or disability requirements. Medicaid and Medicare application information can be found at your state's Medicaid office (see www.medicaid.gov) or at the federal Centers for Medicare and Medicaid Services (CMS) Web site (www.cms.gov).

Whether or not adult children qualify for CMS services, their children may qualify for the Children's Health Insurance Program (CHIP). This federal and state–funded and state-administered program provides comprehensive health insurance for uninsured children younger than 18 years old. Income requirements can be less stringent than with Medicaid. Enrollment fees and co-pays are based on family income. Ensuring that your adult child's own children have insurance coverage can lift some of the financial burden of your child's illness (CMS, n.d.).

## Permanent Disability

If your adult child is permanently disabled, he or she may qualify for Supplemental Security Income or SSI. Determination of disability is required, so your child will need to discuss this with his or her physician before applying. Application may be made at a Social Security Office or online at www.ssa.gov/pgm/ssi.htm.

## Leave From Work

You, your adult child, and your child's spouse may be eligible to take time off work for illness-related reasons without risk of job loss.

The Family and Medical Leave Act (FMLA) entitles eligible employees of companies that have 50 or more employees to take time off to manage healthcare issues, such as therapies, physician visits, and hospitalizations. The employee must have worked for the company more than one year. Health care must be continuous, and leave can be taken in blocks of time. The company must continue to provide group health insurance coverage under the same terms and conditions as if the employee had not taken leave. Eligible employees are entitled to 12 work weeks of leave every 12 months for a variety of reasons including to care for the employee's spouse, child, or parent who has a serious health condition or if the employee has a serious health condition that makes the employee unable to perform the essential functions of his or her job. The employer's human resources representative must be contacted to apply and physician verification is required to prevent fraud (U.S. Department of Labor Wage and Hour Division, n.d.).

The Americans with Disabilities Act (ADA) prevents job loss from calling in sick due to serious illness, such as cancer. The ADA also has a provision that requires reasonable accommodation for chronic illness and disabilities. Encourage your adult child to tell his or her supervisor about the illness and the need to have flexible hours or "flex time." Physician verification of need will be required to prevent fraud (U.S. Equal Employment Opportunity Commission, 2002).

## The Military

If your child is a member of the armed services or a veteran, the FMLA may apply as well. FMLA may be requested if your adult child meets certain active duty requirements. If your adult child is a veteran or service member, your adult child's spouse, son, daughter, or parent may request up to 26 work weeks of leave during a 12-month period to care for the veteran or service member. The employer's human resources representative must be contacted to apply and physician verification is required to prevent fraud.

If your child or child's spouse is a veteran and requires the regular attendance of another person to perform activities of daily living, the Veteran Aid and Attendance or "A&A Pension" may provide help. A veteran's ill spouse also qualifies for services (VeteranAid.org, n.d.).

Information about veterans' benefits may be found at your regional Veterans Service Organization. Determining eligibility and completing applications can be daunting. The application alone is 64 pages long. Trained counselors, many of them retired military members, are available to offer guidance in obtaining services.

# Healthcare Reform

No discussion of healthcare provision and healthcare financing would be complete without a brief discussion of the Patient Protection and Affordable Care Act signed into law in 2010. Also called Health Care Reform, the Affordable Care Act (ACA), and ObamaCare, it is a massive attempt to overhaul the very expensive and fragmented healthcare system in the United States. To say that this law is a work in progress is a vast understatement. At the time of this writing, the Supreme Court recently determined whether one of the foundational requirements in the law is even permitted under the United States Constitution. This requirement is called the "individual mandate" and requires every person in the country to pay for basic healthcare insurance or pay a penalty. Most of the major provisions of the law are not scheduled to take effect until 2014 or later.

Briefly, the ACA focuses on three aspects of health care: cost, access, and quality. It requires private insurance companies to offer coverage to people with preexisting conditions, allows parents to keep adult children on their policies until the child's 26th birthday, and opens health insurance options to new patients. The ACA provides incentives to develop higher quality, more cost-effective methods of delivery of care. The full law can be found online, as well as frequently updated sections describing key features and timelines for implementation (U.S. Department of Health and Human Services, n.d.).

## Advocates

The healthcare system in the United States has many layers. Each layer has its own set of helpful resources and confusing rules. The discussion in this chapter is a brief introduction to get you started to become a source of good information for your ill adult child. You may find that your child needs specific individualized information.

Each bill received from physicians, laboratories, pharmacies, and hospitals should be carefully reviewed. Bills should list each item that was charged to your child or his insurance. If he did not receive an itemized bill, call the organization's billing department and ask for one. He should question items on the bills that he does not understand or which do not seem legitimate to him. This is a good example of how you can help. With your child's written permission, you can make these calls for him. If the insurance company does not cover the entire bill and you and your child don't understand why, call. Be sure to have the insurance policy number available for quick reference.

From time to time the insurance companies' or healthcare providers' reasoning may seem flawed to you. Examples abound of inconsistent logic used by insurance companies to refuse payment for one part of treatment but not others. Danielle told of her insurance company covering a preoperative physical examination, but refusing to cover the surgery. Pam related that her insurance company covered a specialized CyberKnife surgery costing over $100,000, but refused to cover the services of the physician who performed the surgery. You may ask why would a preoperative examination be performed if there was to be no surgery, and who was to perform a very specialized surgery if not a surgeon? All insurance companies and healthcare organizations offer appeals processes to help address actual or potential coverage issues. You can get information about the appeals process in the policy or by calling the organization and asking for the person who handles appeals. In any instance where, after a good faith effort to understand your bill, you believe an error has been made, your adult child should consider appealing the organization's decision.

The best information about health resources is received when requests are clearly stated. You want to be sure that the people you contact understand your request and feel as though their time was well spent helping you. As you encounter different resources, three phrases will always be helpful:

• "I need your advice." This phrase will focus the conversation around the issue you want to discuss. Prepare your request beforehand so that you can explain what information you need. Be clear about what you don't understand and what information you are seeking. "I need your advice" respects the time and expertise of the person you are asking to guide you. You are more likely to get good information.

- "Thank you for sharing your time and knowledge with me." This phrase will keep the door open to future requests. Everyone wants to feel valued. This phrase will convey your appreciation to the person who helped you learn what you need to know.
- "Is there anyone else that you think I should also talk to?" People working in health care have a vast amount of knowledge of healthcare services. Sometimes just asking this question will trigger an idea, a person's name, or another way to think about a tough issue.
- Additionally, you may want to ask, "Do you know if a case manager, patient navigator, or patient advocate is available to help me?"

As noted previously, a case manager from your insurance provider can help you understand the services covered by your policy. Case managers may also work in hospital settings. Often these professionals are experienced nurses or social workers whose job is to help patients and their families get the help they need to be discharged from the hospital to the right level of care at home or in a rehabilitation facility.

A relatively new service provided by healthcare organizations is called a *patient advocate* or *patient navigator*. These positions are typically held by experienced registered nurses or social workers. Patient advocates and navigators work with patients who have complex illnesses and their families to help them ask the right questions and obtain the right information in a way that is understandable. Your physician or hospital nurse may know if this is available for your adult child's condition. Patient advocate services are also available as private services offering information and direct advocacy (Cancer*Care*, 2012; Canosa, 2010).

# Fund-Raisers

Fund-raisers are a popular way to raise money for medical expenses. Fund-raisers can take many forms: selling items, such as candles or candy, and sharing the profits with a supplier, or raising funds through food, such as a dinner or a bake sale where participants pay an amount that covers the cost of the food (if the food is not donated) plus additional money to be given to the recipient. Raffles, garage sales, marathons, dance-athons, and auctions (silent and otherwise) can be used to raise funds for a cause. Often, local businesses, such as restaurants, bars, ice cream parlors, and hair salons, are willing to set aside a block of time where all or a portion of their earnings for that time go to a specific cause. The list of events that can be used to collect donations from concerned individuals is almost endless. It can be done entirely online through social media channels. Fund-raising can be done with the services of a formal fund-raiser or with the commitment of a group of good friends. Fund-raising can be profitable and affirming for the individual.

Fund-raising is also very hard work. Constant communication with possible donors is essential for success. Communication can be very grassroots, such as flyers placed at church or the workplace, or more formal, such as a printed invitation to a gala. Communication can be virtual and potentially very far reaching such as through Facebook, Twitter, Google+, or other social media. To be successful, though, communication has to be frequent, repetitive, clear, and appealing.

Financial rules about fund-raising are complicated. It is not possible to simply raise money and hand it over to a deserving individual. Money raised may be subject to income tax. You must be able to prove that the money raised for a specific purpose was indeed used for that purpose. If you are the fund-raiser, the money you raise must be kept in a separate account. Expenses must be carefully tracked. Fund-raising takes time and skill.

If you are considering fund-raising to help your ill adult child with healthcare-related expenses, talk with professional fund-raisers and get the advice of a tax attorney or accountant. Careful planning will allow a fund-raiser to lighten the costly burden of illness, not add to its financial headaches.

## When Knowledge Isn't Enough: Deciding to Give Money

The decision to give or loan money to adult children is not an easy one. Very few are wealthy enough to give away money without consideration of future consequences. Even for people with similar assets, there is no one right answer to the question: Should I give money to my ill adult child? The knee-jerk or impulsive answer might be "Absolutely yes!" or "No, never!"

Yet, you are encouraged to think through money-related decisions before reaching for your checkbook or liquidating retirement assets. Your goal in giving or loaning money to adult children is to help, not enable them. Even if you are as rich as Warren Buffet, you should not say yes right away, advises Nolan Baker, a financial consultant. Sit down together and have the very hard conversation. Establish boundaries. If you choose to give or loan money, let your adult child know that you are happy to be able to help now, but may not be able to continue to do so in the future. Most adult children do not want to jeopardize their parents' future. Most adult children want to provide for themselves and are reluctant to be placed back in the position of a dependent child. Both you and your adult child should agree to be honest and respectful, not patronizing or condescending during all parts of this ongoing conversation.

Think about how this decision relates to your personal financial stability as well as your family situation. Decisions can be clearer if the following questions are considered.

## Gift or Loan

Deciding whether to give money as a gift or a loan also requires careful thought. There are good arguments on each side of this question. You will need to make the right decision for you and your family. Here are some advantages and disadvantages of both loaning and giving (also called "gifting") to your ill adult child.

"I advise parents [to] never loan their children money," said Baker. "The most important issue is whether parents can afford to part with their money without jeopardizing their present or future stability. Work with a financial expert. Understand the statistical probability of success if you take away the money from your savings. If you can afford to give money, then gift it. The parent-child relationship is a very intimate and fragile one. If a loan is made and the child defaults on the loan, damage to the relationship could be significant. In addition, loaning puts the parent and child in a master-slave relationship. I think of the Biblical teaching in advising against it. A master-slave relationship is not good to have between parent and child" (personal communication, March 13, 2012).

Florida attorney Eric Millhorn (personal communication, March 26, 2012) takes a different view. "Parents who give their adult children money should first consider giving it as a loan," he recommends. "A loan, put in writing, has the advantage of assuring the money goes to the child and is not subject to capture from other creditors that your child may have." Millhorn further points out that if adult children qualify for other benefits, such as Medicaid or SSI, a loan will not penalize them or risk loss of benefits. A loan will also provide some protection to parents in the unfortunate cases where the adult child is not around to pay back the loan.

The decision to loan or gift money to adult children is not a simple one. Certainly, the best advice would be to consult your conscience and a competent tax attorney or financial consultant before making the decision.

## Retirement Savings

Calculating whether you have enough money to give to your ill adult child without affecting your retirement savings can be complicated. It is important to understand your financial plan, explains Baker. Consider tapping into any emergency funds you may have first before you touch retirement savings. You may be subjected to very high penalties if you tap into individual retirement accounts (IRAs) before you are 59½ years old. Furthermore, using retirement savings will decrease your financial return and jeopardize your living standard when you do retire. Completing a Monte Carlo Analysis will help you predict what would happen to your retirement standard of living if you take away a given amount from savings. A Monte Carlo Analysis gives you a statistical probability of successfully meeting your retirement goals if you take away a certain sum of money. Although most people are not familiar with this level of financial planning, "some persons are able to calculate this analysis on their own," explains Baker. "I recommend the MoneyGuidePro (www.moneyguidepro.com) software for those able to do this themselves."

Giving money to your ill adult child could lead to some unanticipated penalties. For example, if you give your adult child a gift that exceeds $13,000, the gift must be declared on that year's income tax filing, notes Millhorn. In addition, if your child receives monetary benefits that are income dependent, such as SSI, a large monetary gift could cause those benefits to be revoked for a time, he advises.

Consequently, if you are giving your adult child money to be used for a specific purpose, such as healthcare expenses, it may be better for you to pay that bill than to give your child the money directly to pay the same debt. In other words, if you pay the hospital bill, you can be sure the money will go where you want it to go and your child will not be penalized.

You could also be penalized if you decide to give money to your ill adult child. Parents may not be aware that transferring money can be viewed as an opportunity to get rid of assets in an attempt to qualify for federal or state benefits. According to Millhorn, even if your intentions are pure, if you intend to apply for Medicaid benefits, there are limits to the amount of money you can give away without affecting your eligibility. For example, if you give away $5,000, you will affect your ability to qualify for Medicaid long-term care payments for one month;

if you give away $20,000, you will affect your eligibility for four months.

Finally, if you choose to loan money to your adult child and your income tax return is audited, you will need to prove you charged at least minimal interest on that loan. A tax accountant or tax attorney can give you advice about this minimal interest rate called *imputed tax rate.*

Your money may be at risk if your child owes creditors for healthcare or other expenses and you have a bank account that is jointly held. Sometimes parents worry about trusted family being able to access financial assets in the case of serious illness and incapacity. To ensure that bills are paid in that event, parents may choose to list an adult child on a bank account. This is a very sensible idea as long as creditors are not trying to locate the adult child's assets in order to pay outstanding debts. In that case, your money in a joint account could be at risk.

## Legacy Money

If you can't afford to give money now, you may be able to provide for your ill adult child when you die. Attorney Mark Clair frequently says, "Be brave enough to face your own mortality and wise enough to do something about it" (personal communication, March 13, 2012).

No matter how much or how little money you believe you will leave when you die, it is best to protect every penny. An attorney or financial consultant can help you leverage what you do have. Leveraging implies using something you have now to increase your financial return at a later time. Life insurance is an example of leveraging a small amount of money into a larger amount. If you qualify for life insurance and can afford the premiums, you may be able to leverage a smaller payment each month for a larger benefit to your adult child when you die.

"If I had to point to one area that almost no one has paid enough attention to, it is the designation of beneficiaries," said Clair. If you have life insurance or retirement accounts or pensions, check to be sure that you have declared the right people to receive your money when you die. "Over half of my clients are shocked to learn that their beneficiaries needed to be updated. Be sure you are providing for those you want to protect when you are no longer here" (personal communication, March 13, 2012). Beneficiaries directly inherit money and are not affected by instructions left in a will or a revocable trust.

An attorney can help you decide whether a will or a revocable trust would be most advantageous for your situation. Basically, a will gives instructions to the probate court about where you want your assets to go when you die. A revocable trust gives instructions to a person who you designate (called a trustee or administrator) to carry out your wishes. Depending on your needs, a trust may give you more flexibility and may save some probate court costs. On the other hand, setting up a trust is more expensive than writing a will and requires more expertise to manage over time. The decision to choose a trust and a will or a will alone can only be properly made after a careful evaluation of your finances, your family's needs, and your wishes.

## Financial Professionals

You are wise to get the advice of financial and legal experts before giving away substantial sums of money. These specialists can help you understand the best ways to protect your assets while maximizing the financial assistance you are able to provide. Again, no matter your financial status, if you have any assets you don't want to lose, such as a house, automobile, retirement accounts, or bank accounts, and want to protect yourself while helping a seriously ill family member, you should seriously consider a consultation with an attorney and a financial professional. Here is a basic overview of what you should expect from these professionals and how to find an expert that is right for you.

Before paying money to any financial or legal advisers, check out their reputation with the Better Business Bureau. Call the bar association in your area and find out if there have been any complaints about the attorney you are thinking of using. Go to the Internet and look for complaints or accolades. If you have homes in two states, such as a winter home in the warmer climates and a summer home in another state, check to be sure that the advice you get from your attorney applies to your state of permanent residency. One of the best ways to learn about an attorney or financial consultant is through word of mouth. Look around at your friends and acquaintances. Which ones seem to be doing well financially? Ask them for a reference. Most people will be pleased that you noticed their financial acumen and will be glad to give you names of those whom they trust with their money and estate planning.

There are three types of professionals who may help you invest your money: insurance licensed professionals, commission-based planners, and financial consultants. Each of them can offer good advice, and each offers a different kind of service. The type you choose will depend on your needs.

Insurance licensed professionals are professionals who sell insurance. While they may have some skills in overall money management, they are not truly financial planners. You do not pay a fee directly to them. They are paid by the insurance companies when you purchase a policy.

Commission-based planners are professionals who sell a financial product or group of products, such as mutual funds, annuities, or stocks. This is the largest group of financial professionals. While their goal is to sell you their products, if their offerings are diverse, they should be able to give you important guidance to choose investments. You do not pay these persons a direct fee. They earn commissions from the products you purchase from them.

Financial consultants are those professionals who will give you advice about a variety of investment options and financial strategies. Their goal is to develop an individualized financial action plan with you. Financial consultants may offer a variety of investment products. Many of their products may be "no load." You do not pay a fee to invest in "no load" products and no commission is paid. You pay a flat fee to a financial consultant for advice, creation of an action plan, and follow-up for a specified period of time.

## Attorneys

Attorneys who specialize in estate law, special needs planning, and elder law are uniquely suited to assist with the legal ramifications of giving money to those you want to protect. Check with your state's bar association to find specialists in your area.

Many attorneys and financial professionals will meet with you for an initial free consultation. During that visit, you should obtain some useful information about the services that are offered by the firm. Both Baker and Millhorn recommend taking advantage of a free consultation. "The match between financial adviser and client is very important since personal information will eventually be shared," said Baker (personal communication, March 13, 2012). "You should leave a free consultation visit with information that can be used, not a sales pitch," said Millhorn (personal communication, March 26, 2012). "Trust is important. If you choose to return to discuss implementing legal protection strategies, then our work can be truly individualized."

## Connie's Story

Fortunately, Mark was surrounded by family and friends well versed in medical care for those without health insurance or the financial means to pay out of pocket for care. Those family and friends helped him to access health care at the price paid by insurance companies and to cover his costs of living. Because he was not able to work during treatment, Mark eventually qualified for his state's Medicaid healthcare coverage designed for low-income individuals. He moved back to his parents' home to decrease rent, utility bills, and food costs.

Mark's story has a happy ending. He has recovered from lymphoma. He completed a Master's in Business Administration and worked abroad for an American bank before returning to the United States and settling in a southern state. He is now a financial analyst, recently married, and happily carrying full health insurance coverage as a benefit of his employment.

# Conclusion

The finances of health care can be formidable. When faced with a request for financial assistance from your ill adult child, take time to gain knowledge about the healthcare system. Learn about benefits that may be available to provide services and financial relief. Use expert help in the form of specialized attorneys, financial professionals, and tax advisers.

It is understandable for parents to want to take care of children, regardless of their age. Thoughtful planning can ensure that you choose the best financial solutions to sustain your financial security while lending a hand to your adult child.

# References

Agency for Healthcare Research and Quality. (2009). *Health care cost and utilization: Statistics on hospital based care in the United States.* Retrieved from http://www.hcup-us.ahrq.gov/reports/factsandfigures/2009/exhibit1_1.jsp

CancerCare. (2012). Financial assistance. Retrieved from http://www.cancercare.org/financial

Canosa, R. (2010). *After treatment ends: Tools for the adult cancer survivor.* New York, NY: CancerCare Inc., Elsevier Oncology.

Centers for Medicare and Medicaid Services. (n.d.). InsureKidsNow.gov. Retrieved from http://www.insurekidsnow.gov/chip/index.html

Patient Protection and Affordable Care Act, 26 U.S.C. § 5000A (2010).

U.S. Department of Health and Human Services. (n.d.). The health care law and you: Key features of the law. Retrieved from http://www.healthcare.gov/law/index.html

U.S. Department of Labor. (n.d.). Health plans & benefits: Continuation of coverage—COBRA. Retrieved from http://www.dol.gov/dol/topic/health-plans/cobra.htm

U.S. Department of Labor Wage and Hour Division. (n.d.). Family and Medical Leave Act. Retrieved from http://www.dol.gov/whd/fmla

U.S. Equal Employment Opportunity Commission. (2002, October 17). Enforcement guidance: Reasonable accommodation and undue hardship under the Americans with Disabilities Act. Retrieved from http://www.eeoc.gov/policy/docs/accommodation.html

VeteranAid.org. (n.d.). The aid & attendance pension. Retrieved from http.//www.veteranaid.org/program.php

**By the Way…**

- Know your role. Most likely, you will be a source of knowledge and information for your adult child. As competent adults, children or their spouses will be talking directly to insurance companies and healthcare providers. You will not.
- Remember that unless you have permission to talk to your adult child's physicians, therapists, hospitals, or health insurance provider, you will not be allowed access to healthcare information. This includes information about billing. Health Insurance Portability and Accountability Act of 1996 (HIPAA) privacy law in the United States is firm and generally well enforced. If your child gives you permission to have access to healthcare information, you must have it in writing. The physician's office, hospital, and state Department of Health may have forms for your adult child to use to grant permission.
- If you cannot find a consent form, see the form in this chapter as an example that could be used for your child to give you access to healthcare and billing information. Remember, if the form is not notarized, healthcare providers and organizations usually will not disclose the information to you.
- Regardless of whether you have permission to directly receive healthcare information, do your homework. Learn how to read a hospital bill. You or your adult child should ask for an itemized bill and look for duplicate charges or charges that seem especially high. Look for the number of hospital days that have been charged. For example, you should not be charged for the day of discharge.
- Learn how to read an estimate of benefits statement from the insurance company. If something seems unclear, call the insurance company and ask to speak to a case manager.
- Negotiate with hospitals and other healthcare providers if your adult child has no insurance and is directly paying for care. Ask for a discount or assistance in working out a payment plan. You have a greater chance for success if you ask before the hospitalization or procedure.
- Hospitals and physicians bill separately. You must negotiate price separately.
- Begin negotiating price with an open-ended statement. Say, "I'd like to talk with you about the hospital cost of my open heart surgery." Avoid saying, "Could I have a discount for my open heart surgery?" The former opens the door to a conversation; the latter often leads to "No." Also, you don't want to say that you want

discount health care. Some providers may interpret this as lower quality care and take offense.

- Physicians and other healthcare providers may be required by insurance companies or office practice policy to try to collect co-pays. Don't ask them to "write off" the charge. They may be prohibited from doing so.
- However, do ask providers if they will accept insurance payment as payment in full. CancerCare has reported success with this approach.
- Talking about healthcare costs is highly stressful. Yet, remember that the person in the billing office did not set the prices you were charged. The amount of your adult child's bill is not her fault. Be courteous when asking for information and seeking clarification. Insulting comments, raised voices, and throwing bills accomplishes little other than making you feel better in the short term; you may well feel childish in the long term. If you need to walk away to calm down, do so. Ask to speak to the person's manager if you or your adult child encounters an impasse.
- If you or your ill adult child believes discrimination has occurred at work because of disability, the Equal Employment Opportunity Commission (EEOC, www.eeoc.gov) may be able to give guidance. The EEOC applies to employees of companies with 15 or more employees (20 or more employees if age discrimination is suspected).
- Consider seeking the advice of a competent attorney and financial consultant who specialize in estate planning, financial planning, and special needs planning. Most good attorneys and financial consultants will offer a free initial consultation. Take advantage of this service.
- The American Cancer Society and the National Endowment for Financial Education have an excellent booklet called How to Find a Financial Professional Sensitive to Cancer Issues. Call the American Cancer Society at 800-227-2345 or go to www.cancer.org to obtain a copy.
- Finding the right financial professional can be done through informal channels such as friends or coworkers or through a financial planning organization. Two examples of such organizations are
  - CFP Board (Certified Financial Planner Board of Standards, Inc.) (800-487-1497, www.cfp.net)
  - National Association of Personal Financial Advisors (800-366-2732, www.napfa.org).
- The Patient Advocate Foundation (800-532-5274 www.patient advocate.org) provides services to patients related to medical debt crisis, insurance access issues, and employment issues for patients with chronic, debilitating, and life-threatening illnesses.

- Many organizations offer discounted services to help ease the financial burden of those with serious or chronic illness. Remember that if you or your adult child are offered a discounted service, a physician's verification of the disability is often required. This is important to prevent fraud. Here are some suggestions.
  - Call your utility company and ask to speak to a service representative about discounts for the disabled. Those discounts often apply to people who must have electricity or gas service at all times directly because of the illness. An example may be the use of a ventilator for breathing. Often such discounts are not well known, so you may need to ask to speak with a manager.
  - If your adult child is not able to dial a telephone because of motor or eyesight problems, some cellular and local telephone services will provide free directory assistance calls.
  - Check with the national organization that supports your child's disease or disability. Often these national organizations have local groups that can provide more immediate help. Examples of some of those groups who do an especially good job providing information and support are the Crohn's and Colitis Foundation of America at 800-932-2423 or www.ccfa.org; American Heart Association at 800-242-8721 or www.americanheart.org; and the Susan G. Komen for the Cure at 877-465-6636 or www.komen.org.

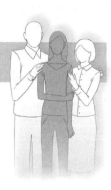

# CHAPTER 6

## THE MEANING OF IT ALL:
# Spirituality

*Make sure you pray when you're well, because when you're real sick, you probably won't.*

—Joseph Cardinal Bernardin

## Catherine's Story

"I t felt like ice water in my veins," said Catherine. "I can feel the shock of learning about Jack's cancer to this day. It was like my circulation froze and then a wave of nausea followed." Catherine is a 59-year-old health professional with an open demeanor and regal bearing. She has decades of experience caring for military veterans. Catherine is no stranger to the effects of war and serious illness on military families.

Yet, when her own adult child became seriously ill she said, "I couldn't make sense of it. How could Jack, my tall athletic 23-year-old, have cancer? He had been tired and a little thin in the fall. But he was starting out in a new business and I thought that normal stress was taking its toll. Then, the last time I saw him, his clothes were hanging off him. I forced him to get the chest x-ray. What more did I miss?"

131

When Jack was admitted to the hospital for surgery to determine the extent of his illness, Catherine remembers praying, "Please let me take his place."

Rather than finding comfort in her professional experience, Catherine recalls, "I was a mess. I started rethinking the importance of everything, my faith, my marriage, my career . . . everything. Nothing was more important than a cure for Jack. I would have traded anything to have him healthy again."

When a child of any age is diagnosed with a serious illness, reactions reach to the depth of a parent's soul. Physical reactions are very common initially. Catherine felt ice water in her veins and nausea.

"When they told me, it was like a spike in my heart," said Addie.

"I became so light-headed, that I couldn't even see the doctor talking to me," said Susan. "I was sure I was dying."

Joan Didion (2011) wrote about feeling a "blinding fury." These parents are telling about a physical reaction to the highly threatening possible loss of their child. The reason for the illness or injury does not make sense. Following bodily reactions come questions that demand a reason. These are questions of the soul.

The question "Why did this happen?" goes unanswered. This cry of the soul is called spiritual pain. Spiritual pain causes suffering.

This chapter will discuss the spiritual pain that comes from feeling the danger of losing your adult child. Spiritual pain and suffering are relieved when a person finds meaning in a distressing situation.

Parents have said repeatedly that faith, hope, and love are needed to recover from spiritual pain. Faith in a power stronger than themselves, hope as a means of increasing confidence, and strength and love as revealed through helping relationships are needed to heal spiritual pain.

What this chapter will not—and cannot—do is tell you exactly what will work to bring meaning to your experience of having a seriously ill adult child. This is highly personal and the authors are not trained theologians or grief counselors. This chapter will share with you what other parents have said about faith, hope, and love so that some light and encouragement may shine on your path.

## Finding Meaning: Faith

When hearing the word *faith*, many think of religion. *Religion* refers to the practice of set rules or dogma within a group of believers. Christianity, Judaism, and Islam are the most common categories of religion in the United States. Hinduism and Buddhism are Eastern religions that are also well represented here. Within these categories are sects, denominations, or subgroups. Christians have many denominations and often call themselves by the name of their group (Roman Catholic, Episcopalian, Evangelist, Lutheran, Methodist, and so on). Jews may identify themselves as Conservative, Reform, or Orthodox. Islam has fewer divisions than Christianity. Most Muslims identify themselves as Sunni; Shia, Ahmadiyya, and Sufi are others.

Religion is important to Americans. A 2011 Gallup Poll showed that 81% of Americans reported religion as "very important" or "fairly important" in their lives. More than 75%

identified themselves as Christian, 2% Jewish, and 7% as "other religion." Fifty-nine percent reported being a member of a church or synagogue. When people were asked how often they attended a faith service, the numbers fell a little. Only 38% reported attending weekly, although more than half, 54%, reported attending a faith service at least monthly. Religion is not seen as perfect by those who responded to the Gallup survey. More than half disagreed with some of their religion's teachings and 25% had switched to different religions as a result of a disagreement with another religion's teachings (Gallup, Inc., 2011).

The Boomer Project, which follows the trends of the baby boomer generation, predicts that as baby boomers age, they will be more likely to regularly attend religious services and turn to help from a higher power. The challenge for this generation is to help answer the question, "What's in it for me?" (Martin, 2011).

Religion is important to us, but belief in God or a Universal Spirit is reported as very important. Whether this unknown source of comfort is called God, Goddess, I Am, Energy Source, Abba, Great Spirit, Allah, or Nature, Americans overwhelmingly believe in a power greater than themselves. In 2011, 92% reported belief in God or a Universal Spirit. In 2007, the last time Gallup asked, 89% believed in heaven and 70% believed in a devil or hell. Belief in something bigger than ourselves is seen as more important than following a set of prescribed religious beliefs. This spiritual side of our human experience brings perspective to our experiences. We look for meaning in bad things through our attention to spirituality.

"Everyone has a sense of spirituality," Chaplain Lee Williams said. "Spirituality is whatever gives us a sense of awe and wonder. Spirituality encompasses our idea of what is perfect. An ill adult child is not right; it is out of order; it is imperfect. We need spirituality to reconcile what is imperfect in our lives" (personal communication, February 26, 2012).

Faith, then, is the ability to see a purpose in a situation and trust that it will turn out the way it is supposed to. Faith allows us to face adversity with trust of help in times of trouble.

"Faith is being sure of what we hope for and certain of what we do not see" (Hebrews 11:1 New International Version [NIV]). Faith offers a gift: peace (Bernardin, 1997).

Catherine, Addie, and Susan related that their first reaction to the shocking news about their adult child's illness was purely physical. Then, the search for meaning in this situation is a search for acceptance. "Why is this happening?" "Why is this happening to my child and not me?" "What is the meaning of this?" "Is this happening because I was a bad parent?" are questions that are answered spiritually, not through reason or feelings.

Sr. Maxine Young said it well: "When such a life-altering situation happens, we have to weave its meaning into our daily life. We need to believe that our experiences mean something important" (personal communication, January 17, 2012).

Finding peace through faith is not simple. Faith, even for those who identify themselves as believers in God or a Higher Power, is not automatic or easy.

"I was suffering," said Donna. "Every day, I would put on a smile and take care of my daughter's children and her house. I would try to do what she and her young family needed. But I couldn't remember the last time I found anything fun. I couldn't just be silly, even with the grandchildren."

"I was so angry with God," said Catherine. "I didn't go to church for a very long time."

"I went to Mass every day," said Eileen, "but I didn't understand why God was making my family suffer."

Suffering is a human response to anguish. There are many definitions of suffering from the most academic to those only worthy of greeting card clichés.

Suffering can be physical, as when bodily pain is experienced. Damage to the body from physical pain usually has an underlying cause, such as a disease. Physical suffering can be visible to others and can be quantified. For example, physical pain can be rated on a scale from 1 to 10. Physical suffering has known treatments, such as analgesics. When physical pain stops, physical suffering stops.

Spiritual pain and suffering is different in important ways from physical suffering. Spiritual pain and suffering cannot be seen by others. Damage to the body from spiritual pain and suffering is not directly caused by a disease or injury, but rather the response to the distressing situation. Spiritual pain and suffering is difficult to define. This is because spiritual pain and suffering refers to any experience that affects a person's core sense of self. In suffering, a person's perception of what is true and valuable is altered. Suffering occurs when we believe that any part of ourselves is at risk of being destroyed and *continues until the threat passes*. When we suffer, we are threatened by future events. What is happening now has frightening consequences for the future.

Theologians use the word *tribulation* to describe suffering and anguish. Tribulation comes from the Hebrew word *tsara* meaning "narrow" or "compressed." The Latin term *tribulum* means a threshing sledge. A threshing sledge is used to separate grain. Suffering or tribulation, then, causes a pressing down or beating as with a sharp heavy instrument. Any of us who have suffered can relate to the sense of being compressed by distress or sharply torn apart by trouble ("Tribulation," n.d.).

All known religions teach that every person suffers. Even devout believers are not exempt from suffering. "He (God) causes his sun to rise on the evil and the good and sends rain to the righteous and the unrighteous" (Matthew 5:45, NIV).

The book of Job in the Old Testament describes a man of strong faith who lost literally everything he owned and loved (Job, 1–42, NIV). Job's faith remained strong until the very end when he had nothing left and even his friends were no help. Job finally gave up, began complaining freely about the unfairness of his situation, and yelled at God. In the end, Job accepts his suffering and all his belongings and loved ones are restored to him many times over.

Some religions teach that suffering is God's punishment for sins. Suffering people struggle to understand God's purpose in causing this suffering and to accept the promise of peace during tribulation. Suffering is explained by some religions as work of the devil or Satan. Conversely, suffering may be seen as a way a loving God tests the strength of the faithful so that spiritual growth can occur.

Suffering is terrible. It can threaten to ruin the sense of what is good. Many would say that trying to find a good reason why people suffer is a futile human effort.

Rabbi Marc Gellman (2012) has said that suffering is a mystery, not a problem with an answer. There is no answer to why people suffer like there is an answer to a multiplication problem. Looking for hidden meanings about why things happen doesn't help suffering. Platitudes, even from well-meaning friends, don't help. Suffering is awful and tears us apart.

The actual or potential fear of losing a loved one causes intense spiritual pain and suffering. Parents say that suffering is intensified when the fear of loss involves a child of any age.

"I felt so guilty. I couldn't shake the feeling it was somehow my fault," said Elaine.

"I don't know of anyone who could cause me such pain other than my child," said Addie.

Nearly every parent said, "I wish it was me. I would trade places with him in a moment." Don Piper, a clergyman who was seriously injured in a motor vehicle crash, wrote, "My dad told me, 'I would give anything to trade places with you and take this on me,' I realized then how much my dad loved me" (Piper & Murphey, 2004, p. 102).

People who turned to their faith during times of family member illness reported fewer stress-related illnesses (Ferrell & Coyle, 2008). "I used my faith and prayer to keep the anger away," said Susan. "When she was sick, I felt like I lost control of everything. Crying to God helped me."

"My pockets were empty; my hands were empty. I couldn't keep fighting my daughter's illness. It was only when I stopped asking why was this happening and started asking how can I do this, that I started to sleep better and eat again and feel better," said Addie.

Not all spirituality is an experience with God or an unseen deity. The presence of a higher power can take various forms. "Just going outside helps," said Carole, a chaplain and former oncology nurse. "Spirituality is an awareness of what is holy. Nature shows us what is awesome. Sunshine or thunderstorms or plants or bird songs all speak to our hearts when we're frightened."

Parents who turned to spirituality reported higher levels of acceptance and eventual healing. Prayer was important.

"I prayed every day for her to be made well," said Eileen.

"I prayed for acceptance," said Addie.

"I changed churches and found that I was able to calm down and accept what was happening," said Catherine.

Prayer is a mental activity that acknowledges a relationship between people and their God. In traditional religions, prayer is based on petitions to God for help or acknowledgment of gratitude for good things. Meditation is also a form of prayer. Meditation is a deep reflection on the meaning of life experience. Meditation also involves creativity, search for harmony in the universe, and an appreciation of others. Some Christians have called this "listening to God."

"Finding meaning through God can be difficult. Answers don't come in a loud voice or a crystal clear sign," said Chaplain Kathy Clapp. "Meditating or deeply thinking to consider what God is trying to show you has been helpful to those parents I've worked with. Many have told me that when prayer is coupled with listening, then peace comes" (personal communication, November 1, 2011).

Meaning needs to be explored in all ways that make sense to you. Viktor Frankl wrote of his experiences in Nazi war camps. He said, "Man is not destroyed by suffering; he is destroyed by suffering without meaning" (Frankl, 1946, p. 135). Faith in a spiritual source of peace that is stronger than yourself may help you discover meaning and comfort in an experience that is impossible to fully understand.

## The Strength to Go On: Hope

Hope can bring confidence to coping with a life-altering experience. When a good outcome is not certain, hope can step in. Hope, like faith, is also difficult to explain.

It is easiest to describe what hope is not. Parents who have experienced a seriously ill child, as well as healthcare providers who care for the very ill and dying, remind us that hope is not the same as wishful thinking. Hope is not thinking hard enough to make a miracle happen. Hope is not the same as looking on the bright side. Hope is not lighting enough candles or attending enough fund-raisers or going to church enough. Hope does not come to those who have good-enough faith in God. Refusing to hear about a poor diagnosis or insisting that all medical technologies be used when the prognosis is grim is not hope. Hope is not necessarily happy.

Sometimes when the loss of an adult child is so overwhelmingly frightening, it is tempting to test or dare God to do what we think is best. Some may say "God will provide a miracle if we don't lose hope." Accepting reality can hurt so much that preschool-like thinking can be confused with mature faith. Preschoolers say, "If I really believe in Santa Claus and tell him what I want for Christmas, I will get it." When fear is so strong, some may say, "If I just believe hard enough and ask for a miracle, I will get exactly what I ask for." But disappointment will result at least some of the time when thinking like this. Yet, child-like thinking does not always mean that hope is weak or unfocused.

Hope in its fullest sense was beautifully described by Vaclav Havel (1990): "Hope is definitely not the same thing as optimism. It is not the conviction that something will turn out well, but the certainty that something makes sense, regardless of how it turns out" (p. 180). Some parents have said that hope is believing things are turning out the way they are supposed to and that they have been given the strength to handle or cope with the outcome.

The parable of the dandelion illustrates this. A man with great pride in his lawn found himself with a large crop of dandelions. He tried everything he could think of or read about to get rid of them. Finally, he wrote to the Department of Agriculture and told them everything he did. The reply came back after a while: "We suggest you learn to love them."

When a child is very ill and the prognosis is unknown, what parents hope for can change and can change often. At the beginning of the illness, hope is for a cure. As a condition becomes more chronic, we may hope for our child's ability to carry out life's tasks or for diminished pain. We may hope not that the intestinal disease is healed, but that our child can learn to live a good life with a colostomy (Puchalski, 2001).

"I have learned that the 'line in the sand' changes," said Delores, a hospice counselor. "I'm often surprised at how people adapt to things they said they would never tolerate. Hope means different things during stages of an illness."

Henri Nouwen (1972, p. 77), a theologian, expressed his view of hope in a poem.

> *Hope means to keep living*
> *amid desperation*

*and to keep humming*
*in the darkness.*
*Hope is knowing that there is love,*
*it is trust in tomorrow*
*it is falling asleep*
*and waking again*
*when the sun rises.*
*In the midst of a gale at sea,*
*it is to discover land.*
*In the eyes of another*
*it is to see that he understands you.*

## All That Is Kind, Compassionate, and Helpful: Love

Sr. Maxine Young said, "In the middle of the night, when worrying won't quit, it doesn't really matter why suffering occurs" (personal communication, January 17, 2012). Suffering is dreadful. Everyone suffers. The devout believer, the atheist, and the person who only shows up at church or synagogue for Christmas and Easter or Passover all are likely to experience life-altering events. Suffering threatens to extinguish both faith and hope. Piety doesn't help; platitudes don't help. What does help is love.

Faith and hope are best supported within relationships. Faith and hope are strengthened by those who care.

"Be sure to build your support systems before the crisis strikes because you're going to need them when everything seems out of control," said Hannah.

"It was my relationship with God and my prayer group that has helped me all these years," said Addie.

Those for whom taking care of others comes naturally may see themselves as fixers. They are the first ones on the scene with a casserole and a sympathetic ear. They know what to do to help.

As this chapter has pointed out, though, caregiving can take a toll on faith and hope. Those who give faith and hope to others need support too. Caregiving can be tiring to the point of exhaustion. Help is needed.

Help and support come through love. Love helps make faith visible. Love buoys hope. Love is the only thing that heals the wounds from loss. It can be found in relationships with friends, through creative expression, and through relationships with a divine power.

The Story of the Long Spoons illustrates how friends and family can make the difference between heaven and hell. A woman worked all her life to do what was good and was granted one wish. Before I die, let me see Heaven and Hell, she asked an angel.

The woman was transported to a large banquet hall where tables were piled high with wonderful food and drink. People sat around the tables. Yet everyone looked miserable. Attached to everyone's arms at the elbow were spoons made of the finest silver. Yet, no one could bend their elbows to eat. Everyone went hungry. This was Hell.

The angel next took the woman to another large banquet hall where tables were again piled with the best food and drink. People sat around those tables as well. Attached to everyone's arms at the elbow were silver spoons. But everyone was happy and content. "What is the difference?" asked the woman.

"Look," said the angel. "These people have learned to feed each other."

The difference between Heaven and Hell is the ability to give and accept help from one another (Enquire Within, 2012).

Friends, especially close friends, can be invaluable in helping to accept the difficulties of an ill adult child. Yet, offers to help are often resisted.

Can you relate to any of these statements?

- "I don't want to bother other people."
- "I'm too busy to ask for help."
- "I ought to be able to cope; after all, he is my child."
- "I don't want to be a whiner. People are annoyed by whiners."
- "When people say 'how are you?' I always say 'fine' because that's what they want to hear."
- "I get tired of hearing the same old complaints in my head all day. Who would want to listen to that?"

Don Piper tells how he kept those who wanted to help him at a distance. He reasoned that no one wanted to be burdened with his suffering. He admits he missed the point: in allowing others to help him, he gave them a chance to find satisfaction (Piper & Murphey, 2004). As we care for others, it is good to allow others to care for us.

Simply sharing the experience with a trusted friend develops resiliency. Being listened to is a sign of love and care. We can bounce back quicker when we understand how normal our situation really is. "I had to learn a new normal," said Catherine. "I really think that my friends from work helped me become more durable and strong."

"You have to remake your edges so you fit," said Darlene. "My friends and my work at the cancer prosthetic shop helped me become OK again."

Catherine and Darlene are describing resiliency.

When people are suffering, there is very little that truly helps other than to be present. Efforts at getting day-to-day things finished are part of this. The little things make a difference: mowing the lawn and making dinner. For those who don't have the time or skill to cook, offering to walk the dog or giving a gift card to a local restaurant that offers both sit-down and carry-out options can be helpful. Being there dependably is a sign of love. The steady presence of a caring person gives strength to keep on going.

"If I'm a mess, I'm no help to Mandy," Susan said. "If I get sick from having no support for myself, then I lose control of everything."

"It is all about the support," said Donna. "My friends made me feel like I'm lucky and can cope."

"I know it sounds corny, but it's true. My friends have been a visible sign of the divine," said Addie.

Creativity is another way to show love. Creating something is in direct contrast to loss. Creativity can take many forms and work with almost any medium: paint, pottery, yarn, fabric, and living plants to name a few.

Creativity is therapeutic in two main ways. First, the energy used to make a work of art or plant a garden or build a model can redirect anger, worry, and fear. Creative energy clears thinking. Second, creation is a defiant act toward illness. If something is being built or made, then a measure of control over the destruction of sickness is achieved.

"I can't paint or do crafty things," said Maggie. "But I can make wonderful pastry. My neighbors all benefit from my cookies and pies when I am trying to work out my anxiety about Sean's heart problems!"

Addie said that the love of friends and appreciation of nature and beautiful things is a visible sign of divine love. Divine love is the love that comes from a higher power or God. Unlike friends, family, and nature, divine love is perfect, fully accepting and forgiving.

The presence of a sustaining, all-powerful God is a great comfort to many parents of ill adult children. Knowing that friends and family were praying for him reminded Cardinal Bernardin of a community of hope.

Believing that nothing can happen that will break the love or connection with divine love gives confidence. This connection is often referred to in terms of a relationship with God and increases hope.

"When my friends and family just didn't get it, praying to God gave me strength," said Susan.

"I prayed that my nourishment would go to my daughter and I would find enough nourishment in God," said Addie.

"God is big enough to handle your anger and fear," Chaplain Lee Williams tells parents and patients (personal communication, January 12, 2012). "You can't break God. God is love."

## Catherine's Story

Jack's illness created a spiritual crisis for his mother. "I'm glad I took advantage of the medical experts I knew from my work," said Catherine. "But I needed more. I looked for direction and found it in unexpected places. I found myself drawn to those who could support me . . . friends, physicians, chaplains. I zeroed in only on what could bring me strength and healing. For the first time, I felt close to God. I was visited by the Blessed Mother who gave me such hope." Unfortunately, these spiritual changes in Catherine were unacceptable to her husband. They separated and later divorced. Catherine left her mainline church and joined a small church in her neighborhood.

Today, Jack's illness is in remission. Catherine continues to be active in her church and find strength in her faith. She continues to see signs of God's love and intervention in her life. "It's like I found clarity. The people from my church surrounded me with love and support. They helped me see that I had what I needed to get through that awful time."

## Conclusion

The message is clear. Spirituality is part of all of us. It is spirituality that allows us to make sense of life experience, have confidence we can cope with whatever happens, and know that our lives are part of something powerful and ultimately good.

Let others help, create something from the energy of your worries, and focus some time each day considering a power greater than yourself. "And now these three remain: faith, hope and love. But the greatest of these is love" (I Corinthians 13:13, NIV).

**Beatitudes for Carers**

A *beatitude* is a supreme blessing for happiness found in heaven. Beatitudes describe happiness not from earthly riches, but from the milk of human kindness. The following are beatitudes written especially for caregivers by an unknown author.

Blessed are those who are gentle and patient—
    for they will help people grow as the sun helps the buds to open and blossom.
Blessed are those who have the ability to listen—
    for they will lighten many a burden.
Blessed are those who know how and when to let go—
    for they will have the joy of seeing people find themselves.
Blessed are those who, when nothing can be done or said, do not walk away but remain a comforting and supportive presence—
    for they will help the sufferer bear the unbearable.
Blessed are those who recognize their own need to receive and receive with graciousness—
    for they will be able to give all the better.
Blessed are those who give without hope of return—
    for they will give people an example of God.

*Note.* Based on information from Bilyk, 2008; Lane, n.d.

# References

Bernardin, J. (1997). *The gift of peace.* New York, NY: Images Books/Double-day.

Bilyk, M.K. (2008, December 20). Beatitudes for caregivers. Retrieved from http://www.marciabilyk.com/2008/12/beatitudes-for-caregivers.html

Didion, J. (2011). *Blue nights.* New York, NY: Knopf.

Enquire Within. (2012, February 11). Allegory of the long spoons. Retrieved from http://whatarewegunnado.blogspot.com/2012/02/allegory-of-long -spoons.html

Ferrell, B.R., & Coyle, N. (2008). *The nature of suffering and the goals of nursing.* New York, NY: Oxford University Press.

Frankl, V.E. (1946). *Man's search for meaning.* New York, NY: Simon & Schuster.

Gallup, Inc. (2011). Religion 1992–2011. Retrieved from http://www.gallup. com/poll/1690/religion.aspx

Gellman, M. (2012, February 9). Suffering is a mystery, not a problem. *God Squad*. Retrieved from http://www.arcamax.com/religionandspirituality/ godsquad/s-1093949

Havel, V. (1990). *Disturbing the peace*. New York, NY: Vintage Books.

Lane, T. (n.d.). Homily for the fifteenth Sunday of year C. Retrieved from http://www.frtommylane.com/homilies/year_c/15.htm#beatitudes_for_ carers

Martin, J.W. (2011, December 31). 10 ways boomers will transform 2012. *Richmond Times-Dispatch*, p. A9. Retrieved from http://www.boomerproject .com/documents/viva/10_Ways_Boomers_Will_Transform_2012.pdf

Nouwen, H.J.M. (1972). *With open hands*. Notre Dame, IN: Ave Maria Press.

Piper, D., & Murphey, C. (2004). *90 minutes in heaven: A true story of death and life*. Grand Rapids, MI: Baker Publishing Group.

Puchalski, C.M. (2001). The role of spirituality in health care. *Baylor University Medical Center Proceedings, 14*, 352–357.

Tribulation. (n.d.). In *Holman Bible Dictionary*. Retrieved from http://www. studylight.org/dic/hbd/view.cgi?number=T6312

## By the Way...

- Everyone has a sense of spirituality. Spirituality is *not* the same as religion. Spirituality *is* a sense of the sacred. Every time you feel a sense of awe, you are experiencing the spiritual side of yourself.
- Let others help you. The presence of others helps validate that your suffering is normal but not deserved or right.
- Carefully choose who you tell very intimate information about your situation. Seek out those who are good listeners and avoid gossipers.
- Talk to other people who are in your situation. Online support is helpful to many.
- To find an online group that has experience with your adult child's disease, go to an Internet search engine* or use the search box located on your Web browser's (Internet Explorer or Firefox, for example) home page. Type in your child's disease and support group. For example, if you are looking for an online support group for those who have diabetes and care for those with diabetes, type "Diabetes: Support Groups" or "Diabetes: Caregivers."
- A free service to support cancer caregivers is found through the 4th Angel Patient and Caregiver Mentoring Program. Scott Hamilton, Olympic figure skating champion, identified three angels who helped him through his treatment for testicular cancer in 1997. Those three angels were his oncology physician, his oncology nurse, and his family and friends. His fourth angel was missing: someone who had gone through the same experience he had, someone who had "been there." The 4th Angel program was created to fulfill this need for others diagnosed with cancer. Mentors for caregivers are available. More information can be found at 216-445-8734 or toll free at 866-520-3197 and online at www.4thangel.org.
- An online site that is specifically designed to help parents of adult children communicate with one another can be found at www.illadultchildren.com.
- Spirituality helps us resolve imperfect things in our lives, such as things that cause suffering to us or to those we love. Exercise helps relieve suffering. Go outside and take a walk, even if just to the end of the driveway and back.
- Consider volunteering with an organization that has helped your adult child. For example, participate in a Walk for the Cure, work in a prosthetic store, or talk to high school students about the importance of breast or testicular self-examination.

- Therapists can help. Do not hesitate to talk to a therapist who specializes in grief and loss. Their input can be very helpful and often in just a few sessions.
- If you feel close to your church and your clergy, speak to him or her. Clergy can often alleviate misunderstandings you may have about God punishing you or your adult child for past misdeeds. Clergy may also be able to put you in touch with small groups at your church who are coping with the same issues you are.
- Spiritual health is closely related to physical well-being. Don't forget to eat and rest. See your physician if you find that poor eating and insomnia are becoming chronic. If you become run down, you will not be able to help your adult child.
- Don't be afraid to laugh. "We used to have inside jokes," said Donna. "If a doctor or a nurse said a certain phrase, we would dissolve in laughter. I'm sure no one would think it was funny but us." "My son's friend used to call him Chemo Sabe," said Katie. "Cancer treatment is so scary that this little joke helped. It still makes me smile."
- Purposefully create. You don't need to be Picasso or The Great Gourmet to benefit. If you can't think of anything you might be good at, investigate your senior center, church, or the adult continuing education offerings from your community college.
- Let go what you can and hold onto what you have to.

*A search engine is designed to search the Internet for topics that are typed into a "Search" box. When you type in the words that you are looking for, the browser will give you all the Web sites found with those words in them. Be creative: type in as many related words as you can think of. Type the words in groups or singly. You won't break the Internet. There are many search engines. Some examples are Google (www.google.com), Yahoo (www.yahoo.com), and Bing (www.bing.com).

# CHAPTER 7

# ARE YOU TALKING TO ME?
# The Right Message in the Right Way

*One of the basic causes for all the trouble in the world today is that people talk too much and think too little. They act too impulsively without thinking.*

—Margaret Chase Smith

## Vanessa's Story

Lauren is a 38-year-old woman in treatment for a multiple sclerosis (MS) flare-up. Lauren was diagnosed with MS a number of years ago. Flare-ups are occurring with increasing frequency. Her mother, Vanessa, is a very organized person who manages a career, marriage to Lauren's father, and involvement in her church. When Lauren is ill, Vanessa helps her son-in-law care for her grandchildren by sharing in carpooling and fixing meals. She has read up on Lauren's condition on the Internet and often updates her daughter about "the latest thinking" on MS. Vanessa describes Lauren as her "best friend." They chat many times each week in person or on the telephone. When she learns that Lauren and her husband are making decisions about medical treatment without her input, she thinks that is wrong and she tells them so. Now, relationships are strained. Vanessa doesn't understand why and is deeply hurt.

# Overview

Communication is well understood as the foundation of relationships. Communication can result in joy and understanding, or anger, hurt feelings, and misunderstanding.

Everyone wants to communicate well. Whole sections of libraries and bookstores are devoted to books telling us how to communicate. Brisk book sales suggest that many people actively seek information and techniques to improve their ability to communicate clearly. Some colleges even offer academic degrees in communications. Whole careers are made from helping others realize how much they need help communicating.

It may seem a logical conclusion that after exposure to so much information and attention, everyone would know how to communicate well in most situations. Yet, especially when the stakes are high, communication often falters. It is tough to master because it always occurs within the circumstances of a relationship. When threatening or frightening events happen within important relationships, ideas and thoughts are not conveyed as well as they could.

It is the meaning of a relationship that makes the outcome of communication important. For example, if the person at the dry cleaners snaps at you and implies you are not very smart when you ask him a question, you may feel peeved, but your self-esteem is most likely not going to suffer and you probably will not dwell on that interaction very long. If your boss or your spouse speaks disrespectfully to you, the stakes are higher, because you probably care more about their relationship with you. Your boss and your spouse are tied to important decisions you have made—your marriage and your job. Criticizing communication with them may make you feel hurt for some time.

The effectiveness of communication between parents and adult children has great consequences. Many parents have said that some of the highest stakes in communication are with adult and nearly adult children.

## Parent-Child Communication

What makes this communication so vulnerable to misunderstanding? Very few relationships are as tied to a person's sense of self as that of a parent to a child. This emotional tie between parents and children spans the child's life. It is reinforced developmentally as parents and children literally mature together. Some experts have suggested that the quality of the relationship with children is intimately related to how well parents think of themselves. If parents think their relationship with their children is positive, then very likely their self-esteem around parenting is strong.

As previously mentioned, the emotional tie is always stronger for the parent than it is for the child. This is particularly true as children reach school age and beyond. Children need parents less than parents need children. From the time a child is a young toddler and can say "I can do this myself," through adulthood, the child's pull toward independence is always stronger than the parental push toward autonomy. Children usually have more confidence in their self-care abilities than parents have in their children's abilities. The turbulent adolescent years are the most obvious example of children's drive to independence in the face of parental caution. Although adult children, especially girls, often move back toward a more positive relationship with parents follow-

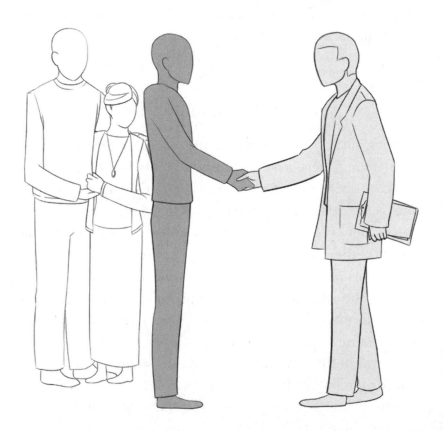

ing adolescence, the child's pull to self-reliance remains part of the relationship. As social researchers Kara Birditt and her colleagues said, "Tensions may be higher for parents than adult children because parents have more invested in the relationship" (Birditt, Miller, Fingerman, & Lefkowitz, 2009, p. 293).

Patterns of adult child–parent communication have been researched. One study of 429 adults conducted by Vital Smarts Research (2005), a corporate training firm, found that 30% of adults say their communication with their parents was less than satisfactory; 33% say they can't spend more than a day with their parents before they feel emotional stress; and 17% say they can't last three hours. A shocking 95% of those who reported a bad relationship with their parents also reported serious illness, whereas only 29% of those with good relationships reported the same (Vital Smarts Research, 2005).

This research is not predictive of every parent–adult child relationship. In fact, researchers from the University of Michigan and Purdue University have shown that adult children and parents tend to try constructive ways to resolve conflict (Birditt, Rott, & Fingerman, 2009). Yet, if even close to one-third of all adults describe a gap in communication with their parents under typical conditions, then how much more stress will serious illness place on communication? Where do parents and adult children go awry? "She had no idea how much we needed her," writes Joan Didion (2011, p. 51). "How could we have so misunderstood one another?"

Parents of seriously ill adult children describe four ideas that seem to influence whether communication with their children will be accepted or misunderstood.

- Having self-awareness
- Respecting boundaries
- Practicing to say it right
- Using information wisely

## Having Self-Awareness

The best way to increase the effectiveness of communication with your adult child is to better understand how your child hears you. If you have not done so, consider thinking about how you are coming across to others. Ask yourself, "Do I seem like a warm human being or a tough-nosed boss?" or "Do I act as though I really want to help or do my offers seem to come with strings attached?" "Do I listen well or is my voice the only one I hear in a conversation?"

Try as hard as you can to not close the door to self-understanding by justifying the way you behave. Your insight will not improve if you begin with thinking, "That nurse is too dumb to understand unless I yell," or "Who does she think she is? I have been his mother for 35 years and she has been around only 10 years," or "If you understood how much this matters to me, then you would understand why I act this way."

If you are having trouble with this self-assessment, ask a trusted friend who will tell you the truth. Consider remembering that this is really not new parenting information. For example, when your children were very young and you were teaching them how to get along with others, your parenting behavior affected how they learned to behave. If you yelled and hit, so did she. If you were calm and talked through your feelings and acted kindly, so did she. This is really not so different. Make sure what you are doing speaks loudly about your love and concern and desire to help, not disrespect of your adult child and her world.

## Respecting Boundaries

Some parents have said that before their adult children became seriously ill, they were convinced their relationship with them was on equal footing. Many parents describe their relationship with adult children as something like a friend. Some parents and adult children even call one another their "best friend." Yet, in every case, this was before the child became seriously ill. Then, as Sharon says, "the Mom Mode kicked in." The desire to protect was stronger than the need to be a friend, and the desire to be cared for was stronger than the need to be a peer.

Obviously, an adult child doesn't need or want his mommy telling him what to do. Protecting and caring for an ill adult child means different things than protecting and caring for a minor child. Things changed in your relationship when your child grew up. Simply going back to what worked when the child was young will almost always result in misunderstanding.

Boundaries between the parents and child change as the child matures. Boundaries change even further when a child becomes an adult and then becomes seriously ill. The pull toward independence and the opposing desire to be cared for as a dependent require new skills for both parent and adult child.

Parents have said that hard lessons were learned about how their adult child wanted help from a parent. Getting used to not being the first person to know everything was an adjustment. Even understanding that legally parents may no longer be the next of kin and receive all health information is easier said than accepted. Asking for permission to help and deferring to a spouse were essential, but not always the first approach parents thought to use.

Many seriously ill adult children reported feeling resentful when their parents treated them "like a child." Some adult children admitted that they shared the good things about their recovery with friends and spouses while only giving minor details to parents. As Liz said, "I love my mom, but when I was diagnosed with breast cancer, I felt like my mom was breathing down my neck. I sometimes shut her out."

Jan, a social worker, intervened between her mother and her seriously ill adult brother. "He wouldn't let her help him with anything. She didn't know how to treat him like a grown-up. I had to talk to each of them so they could learn again how to ask and accept help that worked for both of them."

When adult children are ill, boundaries are often most evident when decisions about communication with healthcare providers are considered. Adult children and parents may have dramatically different ideas about who should be allowed to talk to physicians and nurses, what information is allowed to be shared, and who is included in decision making. Parents have said that learning to respect their child's right to privacy is sometimes difficult. Waiting to receive permission to obtain information is essential.

Parent-child boundaries will always exist. Generational differences, as well as the power imbalance when a child is young, make a truly equal relationship unlikely when the child becomes an adult. For children, it is hard to imagine how the person who told them to pick up their clothes and do their homework and grounded them for unacceptable behavior could ever evolve into a fully equal friendship.

Age and developmental stage will influence just how balanced the relationship becomes when the child becomes an adult, yet adult children and their parents rarely achieve the kind of friendship that is typical of peer adults. In her blog, 40-year-old Jeanne says it well: "Parents need to be the rock you can turn to when you don't know what to do, or when things hurt you or you are in trouble and you don't know how to extract yourself. I'm glad my mom was never my best friend because I love her as my one and only mother" (Kozelek, 2009).

Healthy boundaries help explain why children may look to parents for help and support well into adult years. When she realized that her daughter Hayden was telling her all the bad stuff and sharing the good stuff with other people, Sandy was initially hurt. But then, she said, "You can't worry about whether your child loves you and tells you everything. You are the parent and you are to love your child no matter what."

## Practicing to Say It Right

"Every winter I look forward to watching professional figure skating on television," says Christine. "I reacquaint myself with the proper terms for the skills: axel, butterfly jump, compulsory figures. By the end of an afternoon of watching, I can so feel the thrill of figure skating to beautiful music that I am almost convinced that given the proper laces and skating skirt, I too could compete on ice! I would truly love to glide on the ice. I am sure I could do it!

"That, of course, is nonsense . . . made all the more absurd by the fact that I can scarcely walk down a sidewalk in heels higher than 2 inches. Yet, when I watch the experts skate, they make it look so easy! I start to think 'how hard can this be?' Somehow, I am able to block out the years of dedicated practice that makes these performances look so easy. I begin to think that if I want it badly enough, I could do it in short order."

It is easy to expect that pure desire to perform a difficult skill can overcome the appreciation of practice. Some of the most difficult skills, like figure skating, look easy when experts show off the results of years of practice. Experts in any field will tell you that practice means successes and heartbreaking failures, as well as confidence-building acceptance and being passed over. Practice means doing the same thing over and over so that when the stakes are high, your actions will get you the results you want (Gawande, 2002). Communication with adult children is a difficult skill and requires that level of practice. Some would argue that communicating with children of any age is difficult, but that the stakes are highest when children are older and are independent enough to accept or reject parental input without consequence. In other words, when children are adults, you can't make them do what you say. Your approaches to communication determine whether your input is accepted, only tolerated, or worse, simply rejected.

The communication stakes are often perceived to be higher for parents (Fisher, 2011). The outcome of communication with your adult child probably means more to you than to your child because your attachment is usually stronger. If communication goes wrong, you will probably be more bothered by it. Parents tell many stories about communicating with their ill adult children. Sometimes the outcome has been positive, and sometimes parents have been left feeling hurt and confused.

Parents often thought about both the good and the bad communication encounters with their ill adult children and other family members. They said that when they thought before they spoke and practiced what they were going to say, the outcome was always better. Parents said they have found three communication skills that are essential to understanding: soften your approach, use silence and listening, and show up dependably. These approaches apply whether you are communicating with your adult child, your child's spouse or partner, or your child's healthcare providers.

## Soften Your Approach

"I found that if I was tentative, my comments were better received," said Bonnie. Ask permission to help and be open to helping in any way your child needs and you are able.

Try leading with a positive comment. "You are doing so well handling everything you have to do plus medical treatment. Could I help you with picking up the children from soccer practice or make a casserole for your dinner or something else?"

This does not mean that you have to be dishonest or never give your opinion. Your goal will be to say what you mean without being mean. Parenting and communication experts emphasize describing the effect of a situation on you, not blaming the other person. This is called using "I-messages" versus "You-messages" (Dinkmeyer & McKay, 1976).

For example, saying "You don't tell me what is going on with your treatment; how do you suppose that makes me feel?" will be received much differently than if you say "I feel worried when I don't know what the doctor is telling you. Do you think we could talk about what is planned for your treatment?" I-messages lower defensiveness because no one is blamed. I-messages encourage conversation.

"Avoid using the word *but* when offering your suggestions," advises Samantha. Practice saying phrases such as, "Although you may disagree with me, this is what I think."

Paraphrasing can be a very helpful way of checking to be sure you understand what is being said. Paraphrasing is giving the other person your interpretation of what he is telling you. Paraphrasing can focus on how a situation makes your child feel or summarizes the key ideas. Phrases such as "You are exhausted" or "Not having answers is very upsetting" can make your child feel understood. Here is a word of caution: Paraphrasing is different from parroting. Simply repeating back or parroting what was said can have an irritating effect. For example, your child says to you, "The medication makes me so sick that I can't go to work. If I get fired, how will I pay for my health care?" A parroting phrase, "You can't go to work and might get fired," would be less understanding than the paraphrase, "You're scared that you won't be able to keep your job because you're missing so much work."

Don't be fooled into thinking that a soft or tentative approach is synonymous with being a doormat. It does mean that when serious illness occurs everyone is sensitive. Of course you are very worried and may know you have more experience and wisdom. Yet, this combination of fear and arrogance puts you at risk for sending your messages too bluntly and sounding condemning or belittling.

Because of the age and life stage of most parents who experience serious illness in their adult children, communication skills are stronger than they have ever been. Researchers have shown that people who are middle-aged (40–70 years old) have many communication strengths. Middle-aged adults—regardless of gender or socioeconomic status—have more mature coping skills and are more focused on relationships than younger adults. Middle-aged adults are better at bridging conflict and considering other people's needs. Although overt confrontation may occur when very upset, most middle-aged adults are better at controlling negative emotions and are more conciliatory. Family conflict is more easily bridged (Birditt & Fingerman, 2003, 2005; Oatis & McBurney-White, 2009).

"I have to remind myself that my reaction is only that . . . my reaction. When I point out what I find the most troublesome, I try to be kind," said Lori.

Most parents of seriously ill adult children bring maturity and nuance to intense situations. They understand that situations are rarely black and white.

Approaching softly will deliver the intended message. "I love you. I want to help. Please let me help you."

## Use Silence and Listening

Lee remembers when she knew she was talking too much. "Don't say anything until I've finished talking," said her daughter Emma. "I don't need for you to work this out for me. Just listen!"

One of the most difficult communication skills for any parent is to listen and not offer advice. You may remember that interrupting and quizzing and offering unsolicited advice didn't work when your children were younger; it certainly does not work when they are grown.

Everyone is sometimes tempted to set everyone straight. After all, you may reason, I know best. I have the most invested in this child.

Stephanie recalled, "You're afraid. You want information but you're afraid of the information. The hardest thing and the smartest thing to do is to trust your child."

Pam said, "I had to keep telling myself, 'This is not all about you.' She will make the right decision."

Allie said, "She is his wife and I need to respect that. She is scared too."

Silence and listening means that you have faith that your child will do it right. It means offering information kindly and then letting your adult child make the final decision. If you are asked directly for help, give your advice, make sure it is understood, and then accept what your child decides.

Listening is a powerful tool that can address the need for problem resolution and stress release. It is not a "quick fix" tool. Where human behavior is concerned, there are few overnight solutions. However, people have the natural ability to assist each other by listening. When this ability is developed over time, others can be helped to become more resourceful, more able to care effectively, and more self-assured.

When your child talks and you listen with attention, he knows you care. As the listener, you offer no advice, no helpful hints, and no questions to satisfy your own curiosity. You give full attention and respect. By listening, you are showing that you believe that talking things through will help your child sort and learn from his experience (Oatis & McBurney-White, 2009).

Think about the last time someone thoroughly listened to you. When someone is important enough to be listened to, he gains an understanding of what it is like to be respected and supported while clarifying thoughts and showing feelings. Talking things out helps recover the ability to think clearly and make well-thought-out decisions.

This kind of time to think, uninterrupted, about one's problems is an almost unknown commodity. When parents give their adult children a chance to examine their serious illness experience in detail, they become freer to think of new approaches, to problem solve, and to act intentionally when difficult situations arise. Listening is a very purposeful way to assist your adult child to think and learn. When two people are focused on one person's issues, the doubled attention results in strengthened resolve to reconcile problems (Raveis, Pretter, & Careno, 2010).

Listening requires practice to pay attention and not think about what you are going to say next. Start now. Let your child know you are trying to listen more and give advice less. Chances are that both of you will be relieved. It is a lot of pressure to come up with answers for everything, just as it is frustrating to not tell your whole story without hearing the "best" solution. So, relax. Be silent. Listen. Be confident. Your child will make the best decision.

## Show Up Dependably

"Sometimes, I just came and sat with her during the treatments. We didn't talk much. I was just there. I think it helped both of us," Sandy told us.

There will be times when seriously ill adult children will lash out to parents. "My dad, who lives out of town, never visited or called me once when I was in treatment," said Linda. "He did come to town for my cousin's wedding, though. I told him exactly what I thought, but I don't think he understood how much it hurt me. I felt ignored, really."

There will certainly be times when you may feel as though your adult child only wants you around to have someone to ignore or blame. The temptation to stay away may be strong. A word of caution: avoid avoiding as much as you are able. Evading these difficult times can damage the relationship because it can be interpreted as shunning or abandonment.

The steadiness that parents bring to simply and dependably being present can communicate stability more than words. Just like listening, being present can be comforting. Being present conveys an acceptance of your adult child and his circumstances. When your presence can be relied upon, worry about things unforeseen or dreaded can be shared. When you are present, the good and amusing can also be shared.

Combined with a softened approach and a balance between listening and talking, being present communicates respect. Respect opens communication.

# Using Information Wisely, or Not Believing Everything You Are Told or Read (on the Internet)

A vast amount of information is available online discussing virtually every topic in the world through a worldwide collection of computer networks that form the Internet. Information is easily accessible on laptops, e-readers, tablets, and phones. Information is shared by "friends" in social media, through e-mail lists, and through search engines such as Google, Bing, and Yahoo. The largest of these search engines has become a verb for Internet searching. You say you "Googled" it.

But how much of this information can be trusted? Misunderstandings between healthcare providers and patients frequently occur because information found on the Internet does not tell the whole story, is not well understood, or is incorrect altogether.

Evaluating Internet-based resources for health information is important. Information on the Internet is found on Web sites. The World Wide Web, or simply the Web, is a way of packaging information and sending it over the Internet. Information on the Web is put on "sites" that are built on top of the Internet. Just as a train delivers cargo in boxes, so are Web sites the "boxes" that are sent on the Internet "train." Web sites are usually listed like this: www.nameofwebsite.com or www.othername .org.

Finding Web sites is not difficult. A search engine functions like a very fast, very knowledgeable librarian. On a search engine site, simply type in words that describe what you are looking for, such as "diabetes foot care" or "recipes for soft diets." These are called *search words*. Click Enter and a list of Web sites will appear on the screen. Be creative with search words. You cannot break the Internet and can only get more information. You can also find Web sites listed within written materials. For example, a magazine article about dental care may list a Web site discussing screening for oral cancer. You can type that Web site address in your browser (the top bar of your Web page) or in a search box and find the article. Another way to find a Web site is through a "link" found within an online article. The Web site address is highlighted (often blue). If the address is clicked with the mouse, the Web site will open.

Once you have some Web sites to read, you need to decide if the information is appropriate or not. Some Web sites are quite beautifully designed yet may not contain information that is right for you. If you know how to judge the accuracy and usefulness of a Web site, then you will be better able to understand how to tell a good from a fair from a terrible health Web site.

The basics of Web site evaluation are very similar to those you would use to evaluate written materials such as a newspaper or book. You would not dream of accepting or rejecting any pamphlet, article, or even this book without first evaluating it.

The Internet is a valuable place to look for information to help you and your adult child understand medical care and treatment. Your information will be seen as more legitimate if you know how to find clear, specific, and accurate information on the Web, as well as in other written materials.

### Basic Guidelines for Evaluating Web Sites

**WHO?** Who authored the site? Was the author a medical expert? Can you tell if they are experts in this field? Are their credentials listed or do they just tell you that they are skilled? Who sponsored the site? Do you need to buy something from them to get the information you want?

**WHAT?** What is their point of view? What biases do you see in their site? For example, do they tell you that their position is the only and best way or that the vitamins they are selling will cure cancer? Or, is their site balanced with an explanation about different sides to the topic? What is the reason they are publishing this information?

**WHEN?** When was the site published? When was it last updated?

**WHERE?** Where does this information fit into other information you have reviewed on the topic? Are there links or references to other related topics in the Web site? Does the site tell you where and whom to contact for further information?

**HOW?** How can you verify the accuracy of this information? How could you use this information? How could you contact others for further information?

An excellent source of reliable information is the National Institutes of Health (www.nih.gov). You can start here to find information on almost every health topic. For example, if you are interested in managing heart disease, you could visit the National Heart, Lung, and Blood Institute (www.nhlbi.nih.gov). In addition, you can visit the National Library of Medicine's MedlinePlus (www.medlineplus.gov) for dependable information on more than 700 health-related topics. Another organization, WebMD (www.webmd.com), is a reliable source for general health information, disease information, and consumer updates on health trends.

## Vanessa's Story

When Vanessa realized that her approach with Lauren and her husband was not welcome, she decided to soften her approach. She asked Lauren how she could help, and then followed through. Although she is still not directly included in medical discussions, Lauren has asked her to specifically research some information about MS on the Internet. Vanessa admits that learning to accept Lauren's decisions took some effort.

Lauren's illness has brought out protectiveness and a strong feeling of responsibility. "I just wish it was me instead of her. So I barge in and take over. I'm trying though. I've learned if I listen, she tells me more. So I listen. She asks me for my opinion now and sometimes takes my advice. I can't rush in and make it better, so I will walk through the doors she holds open for me."

## Conclusion

Communication is one of life's greatest gifts and one of the most difficult to get right. Taking time to understand your own parental behavior when communicating with your adult child can have a major effect on how your message is received. Appreciating boundaries will allow adult children to accept your caregiving and support as parents, not as friends. Practicing words of support and listening more than talking are harder than it might seem. Remember that it takes more practice than you might think to master something as hard as letting your child know you trust his or her judgment. Finally, parents have said many times that when they carefully read and understand health information and then respectfully offer that information, their contribution is better received. You are a very important support and decision-making consultant to your child, but you are not the person who will speak on your child's behalf without permission.

# References

Birditt, K.S., & Fingerman, K.L. (2003). Age and gender differences in adults' descriptions of emotional reactions to interpersonal problems. *Journals of Gerontology: Series B Psychological Sciences and Social Sciences, 58B,* 237–245. doi:10.1093/geronb/58.4.P237

Birditt, K.S., & Fingerman, K.L. (2005). Do we get better at picking our battles? Age group differences in descriptions of behavioral reactions to interpersonal tensions. *Journals of Gerontology: Series B Psychological Sciences and Social Sciences, 60B,* 121–128. doi:10.1093/geronb/60.3.P121

Birditt, K.S., Miller, L.M., Fingerman, K.L., & Lefkowitz, E.S. (2009). Tensions in the parent and adult child relationship: Links to solidarity and ambivalence. *Psychology and Aging, 24,* 287–295. doi:10.1037/a0015196

Birditt, K.S., Rott, L.M., & Fingerman, K.L. (2009). If you can't say something nice, don't say anything at all: Coping with interpersonal tensions in the parent-child relationship during adulthood. *Journal of Family Psychology, 23,* 769–778. doi:10.1037/a0016486

Didion, J. (2011). *Blue nights.* New York, NY: Alfred A. Knopf.

Dinkmeyer, D., & McKay, G.D. (1976). *Raising a responsible child: How to prepare your child for today's complex world.* New York, NY: Fireside.

Fisher, C.L. (2011). Her pain was my pain: Mothers and daughters sharing the breast cancer journey. In M. Miller-Day (Ed.), *Family communication, connections and health transitions: Going through this together* (pp. 57–76). New York, NY: Peter Lang.

Gawande, A. (2002, January 28). The learning curve. *The New Yorker.* pp. 52–56. Retrieved from http://archives.newyorker.com/?i=2002-01-28#folio=004

Kozelek, J. (2009). Cats with knives: Mama? Retrieved from http://catswithknives.blogspot.com/2010/09/mama.html

Oatis, P., & McBurney-White, B. (2009). *Listening with connection.* Unpublished manuscript.

Raveis, V.H., Pretter, S., & Carrero, M. (2010). "It should have been happening to me": The psychosocial issues older caregiving mothers experience. *Journal of Family Social Work, 13*, 131–148. doi:10.1080/10522150903503002

Vital Smarts Research. (2005). Healthy communication with your parents. Retrieved from http://cms.vitalsmarts.com/d/d/workspace/SpacesStore/f4b1a7ca-08e5-454d-a921-5f2a36846853/Healthy%20Communication%20with%20Your%20Parents%20Summary.pdf?guest=true

### By the Way...

- When offering your opinion, always lead with a positive comment.
- Ask permission to help; ask what your adult child needs and then follow through.
- Honestly say what you mean without being mean.
- Use I-messages to focus on your feelings, not your child's action.
- Listen more; talk less. If your voice is the only one you hear, you are talking too much.
- Communication is very hard when the stakes are high; practice practice, practice.
  - Practice asking, not telling.
  - Practice paraphrasing.
  - Practice listening with attention.
  - Practice until you feel comfortable.
- When paraphrasing and I-messages feel odd, tell your adult child that you are trying to communicate better so you can share what he or she is going through.
- When you have a strong urge to tell others how things should be done, count to 10, 20, or however high is needed for the urge to pass.
- Use a step-by-step approach to evaluating what you find on the Internet. Remind yourself that if something sounds too good to be true or doesn't make sense, you are probably right.

# CHAPTER 8

# WHAT ABOUT ME?
# Caring for Yourself

*I have mixed emotions when I receive Father's Day gifts. I'm glad my children remember me, but I'm disappointed that they actually think I dress that way.*

—Mike Dugan

*I am fairly certain that given a cape and a nice tiara, I could save the world.*

—Leigh Standley

## Julie's Story

Julie is 57 years old. She has been married to her college sweetheart, Joe, for 35 years, and in those 35 years they have had their share of ups and downs. Recent economic difficulties have dealt them the triple hardships of job loss, selling their home in an undervalued real estate market, and living in separate states because of relocations necessitated by all those factors. That is how at the start of 2011 Julie was living in Cleveland, Ohio, and Joe was living in Eugene, Oregon.

Although both are still renting, Joe's income now allows them to maintain these two residences states apart. Julie has taken early retirement and can now afford the luxury of extended visits to the West Coast. They are eager to live together again, but where? The dilemma is that the job is in Oregon but most of their family is in Ohio, and Ohio is home. Within 10 miles of Julie is her first born, Jen, with her husband and 2½-year-old son; her only sister lives a few minutes from her; and her brother and father live an easy two- to three-hour drive away. Where to live? What to do? They continued to weigh the pros and cons and discuss. Then another story started.

As Julie tells it, during the holidays and into the new year, Jen was tired. Of course, she was caring for a busy 2½-year-old, Lucas, an active, good-natured blessing. Jen was also working as a research associate and going to school to complete her PhD in microbiology. Her husband was working as a teacher and also attending graduate school. At 29 years old, they were building their futures. Jen didn't worry about the fatigue and intermittently wondered if she could be pregnant. That was not the plan, but "surprises" happen. Then she noticed some rectal bleeding.

The rectal bleeding required medical attention, and looking for the source of the bleeding included a colonoscopy. Julie remembers, "When I was called back to the recovery area after the colonoscopy, I knew. I knew when I saw the doctor's face." Jen was facing the "less than 1% chance" of a cancer diagnosis. She was facing colorectal cancer.

Julie will never forget the doctor's words: "I'm sorry. I am shocked."

The day they received the diagnosis is still surreal. Driving Jen back home and then waiting with her until her husband,

Andy, and Lucas came home is forever imprinted in her memory. They cried together.

Julie offered to take Lucas home with her for the night. And although she would take him many times over the next months, that night Jen needed to be with her husband and son. This family needed to be together. Julie respected and understood her decision.

Treatment over the next nine months was intense. Radiation therapy, which sometimes left her skin raw with burns around her anus and increased her fatigue; surgery, which left a scar from under her right breast to just above her pubic bone and included a total hysterectomy (the removal of her uterus and ovaries) and partial removal of her colon with an ileostomy to one side; and finally chemotherapy that resulted in hair thinning, nausea, numbness, pain and tingling in her fingers and toes, and even more fatigue.

"The ileostomy was very hard for her. She didn't want to look at it, and she had very poor training in how to care for it. We were on our own. She has adjusted very well to it now, but every time I go shopping I am constantly looking for clothes that she might like and that would be comfortable. I guess I am always thinking of her," Julie says.

Once treatment was completed, the biggest question was still before them: "How successful were the treatments?" Scans to determine this were scheduled within the next two months. No matter the news, her five-year survival rate was predicted to be 65%–70%. "But there is every reason to hope. These [were] only statistics and based on patients who are usually much, much older than Jen," Julie explains.

Throughout the treatments, Julie helped Jen by attending appointments with her, watching Lucas, cleaning their house, laundering their clothes, and doing yard work for them. She says, "This is about Jen, her husband, and her son. I will be there for her but I let Jen and Andy call the shots."

Julie extends the effort for other relationships, too. She does not forget her son-in-law. He also has a difficult time going through this illness. They had dinner together every night that Jen was in the hospital.

Julie and Joe's other child is two years younger, a son. He also recognizes the support he has received from his parents. During his Air Force commissioning ceremony he said, "I have to thank my parents. Even when they didn't always agree with me, they always backed me 100%." Julie and Joe have done this with intention as they relate to their adult children, their spouses, and their grandchildren.

Jen has also thanked Julie and Joe in many ways. Julie's pride in Jen is undiminished, even enhanced through this ordeal. She frequently comments on how strong Jen is. "One of the fallouts of this strength is that people don't know how sick she is. They see she looks OK and think it must not be so bad," says Julie. But like Andy, sometimes she wants to say to them, "Look at her abdomen—the scars, the ileostomy. She has been through hell and back but she keeps going on. Don't confuse strength or resolve with easy."

Julie's trips to Oregon have been severely curtailed; she has not visited for six months. Joe comes to Ohio, but he has been sheltered from some of Jen's worst times. Julie, on the other hand, often takes the brunt of any anger, despair, or frustration. She is frequently in the line of Jen's fire.

When asked, "What is the one best thing she can do for Jen, the one thing any parent can do for an adult child?" Julie answers quickly, "take care of you. I have heart problems and have seen a specialist. I know I have to walk regularly and have lost weight. I have to be healthy to help her."

Years ago Julie watched as her parents lost their oldest son. He died from complications following a prolonged illness. Julie says, "I don't think my mother ever fully recovered."

Is it possible that Julie and her mother suffer from a broken heart? In the past, the effects of chronic stress were considered a "broken heart." Today, broken heart syndrome is recognized as a bona fide medical condition. It is defined as a temporary heart condition brought on by stressful events and is 7.5 times more likely to occur in women (Mayo Clinic, 2011a). A person experiences sudden chest pain and may think she is having a heart attack. Good or bad stress can trigger a rush of adrenaline and other stress hormones that cause the heart's main pumping chamber to enlarge and not function well. The rest of the heart remains normal. This will cause dramatic and serious changes in the heart's rhythm and the release of substances in the blood typically seen with a heart attack but with none of the artery blockages that usually cause one. The symptoms are treatable and temporary. Although neither Julie nor her mother was diagnosed with broken heart syndrome, their adult children being seriously and life-threateningly ill was very stressful.

The purpose of this chapter is to encourage and help you to take care of yourself, physically, emotionally, and spiritually. There is more information on emotional and spiritual care in Chapters 4 and 6. Although often left until last, perhaps this chapter should be first, because as Julie realized, without her own health she could not sustain another person. As another mother explained, "When my daughter was ill, I would wake up early and not be able to go back to sleep. This got me to some very early, early Sunday morning masses and I wondered, 'Are all these people insomniacs?'" Her sleeping difficulties were accompanied by a 20 lb. weight gain in about a year. Now her daughter has recovered, and the mom is sleeping better, but the weight still unhealthily lingers. From these examples this chapter further looks at what is known about who is giving care.

## Caregiving and the Caregiver

In all shapes and sizes, approximately 30–38 million family caregivers in the United States provide care for about 90% of dependent individuals with acute and chronic physical illness, cognitive impairments, and mental health conditions (Mitnick, Leffler, & Hood, 2010). Family caregivers include relatives, partners, friends, and neighbors who assist with activities of daily living and complex healthcare needs that were once the domain of trained hospital personnel. Patients depend on family caregivers for assistance with daily activities, managing complex care, navigating the healthcare system, and communicating with healthcare professionals.

There are no statistics about how many of these family caregivers are parents caring for adult children. It is also not clear how many parents provide care full-time or part-time. Generally speaking, family caregivers receive little training on how to deliver complicated care, are not treated as partners in their loved one's care, and are not encouraged to maintain their own health. Not surprisingly, research shows that family caregivers are at increased risk for health, emotional, financial, and work-related problems. They need help developing the problem-solving, organizational, and communication skills that the situation demands (Pinchot, 2011).

Research supports that the caregiver role is frequently subjugated or seen as not as important as other roles, for example, to that of the "breadwinner." Parents share that when you are a caregiver, there is no time to be ill, certainly not if you are not as seriously ill as your child. But care for oneself must be valued if one is going to be able to physically, emotionally, and spiritually meet the demands of caregiving.

Dr. Anne Grinyer, a medical sociologist at the Institute for Health Research, Lancaster University, has researched the effects of serious illness of a young adult child on the mother's health. She says, "There is a strong cultural assumption in Western society that our children should outlive us, and it is incredibly hard for a parent to see their child predecease them. Often this will cause the mother to ignore early signs and symptoms of illness" (A. Grinyer, personal communication, August 20, 2010). When their children are seriously ill, mothers frequently do not see space for their own illnesses, saying, "I am not as ill as my child." This attitude discounts their health needs. The lack of attention may have serious future consequences for the mother's health, which may extend beyond the child's illness.

Grinyer (2006) recognizes the realities of a very difficult situation. "All families are different and the danger is that you try to come with a motto that says what you should do for everyone." The preexisting family dynamics must be considered. "If there were any cracks beforehand, they are only going to get worse. Life-threatening illness does not make everyone suddenly like each other. It just puts everybody under terrible pressure" (A. Grinyer, personal communication, August 20, 2010).

Referring to both physical and emotional problems, Grinyer advises, "The more honest the communication, the better it is for everyone. Problems arise when everybody is trying to protect everyone else. I think that a climate of openness, honesty, and trust can strengthen all members of the family" (A. Grinyer, personal communication, August 20, 2010).

Through interviews with mothers caring for their adult daughters with breast cancer, medical sociologist and social gerontologist Dr. Victoria Raveis also determined that the diagnosis of breast cancer affected the whole family. The mothers experienced a variety of emotions including shock, denial, anxiety, fear, sadness, distress, and guilt. They also revealed that they often felt more than one emotion simultaneously, such as being frightened, sad, and angry (Raveis, Pretter, & Carrero, 2010).

Another emotional aspect she found was linked to the potential hereditary aspect of breast cancer. Mothers also felt susceptible, vulnerable, and responsible despite the occurrence of the cancer "out of sync" with the usual course of events. That is, it is usually expected that the parent will first develop the cancer, subsequently with children being at risk for its development. Still the mother asked, "Did I cause my daughter's breast cancer?"

Raveis also found some gender differences in the parental response to their daughter's cancer. The mothers tended to care for the daughter, even moving in with the daughter if necessary, whereas when fathers were involved, they tended to care for their own household in the mother's/wife's absence. Fathers kept things running smoothly.

It is clear that there is much going on simultaneously for everyone involved with a serious illness. Dr. Raveis suggests that parents listen to what is said and recognize that things said out of frustration are not reflective of true feelings. Hurtful things may be said even with the best of intentions. The well person must be aware of the bigger picture. Parents who have negative feelings in these difficult situations should be aware that this is normal. Coping for the parents may be enhanced with education, respite care, self-care, and acceptance of the wide range of feelings as normal.

If the daughter's spouse is present, the caregiving roles and responsibilities have to be negotiated with this key relationship in mind. A disease such as cancer necessitates family-centered care. Dr. Raveis said, "The dynamics of the family influence who is also impacted by the care and how everybody's lives might be transformed. That in turn can influence the quality of life that the patient might be having, their willingness to undergo certain types of treatments, and the ability to fully recover or the speed at which they might be recovering" (V. Raveis, personal communication, August 6, 2010). A 10-year breast cancer survivor recalls how her mother helped care for her young children during her doctors' appointments and treatments. She said, "Knowing mom was home with Kyle and Susan let me focus on learning what I needed to do and then following through. It freed me to concentrate and take care of myself." It is important to remember that what is happening in the family affects the care of the patient and that the stress affects everyone.

# Stress and Stress Management

There is "good" stress. This type of stress motivates us to meet a deadline or get things done. Unrelenting, long-term stress can negatively affect physical well-being, emotions, and behavior. Being able to recognize common stress symptoms can help manage them sooner and perhaps better. Research supports that uncontrolled stress contributes to high blood pressure, heart disease, obesity, and diabetes (Mayo Clinic, 2011b).

### Common Effects of Stress

**Physical**
- Headache
- Muscle tension or pain
- Chest pain
- Fatigue
- Change in sex drive
- Stomach upset
- Sleep problems

**Emotional**
- Anxiety
- Restlessness
- Lack of motivation or focus
- Irritability or anger
- Sadness or depression

**Behavioral**
- Overeating or undereating
- Angry outbursts
- Drug or alcohol abuse
- Tobacco use
- Social withdrawal

**A Story of Stress**

A young lady confidently walked around the room while explaining stress management to an audience. She had a raised glass of water, and everyone knew she was going to ask the usual question, "half empty or half full?" She fooled them all by asking, "How heavy is this glass of water?"

Answers called out ranged from 8 oz. to 20 oz.

She replied, "The absolute weight doesn't matter. It depends on how long I hold it. If I hold it for a minute, that's not a problem. If I hold it for an hour, I'll have an ache in my right arm. If I hold it for a day, you'll have to call an ambulance. In each case, it's the same weight, but the longer I hold it, the heavier it becomes."

She continued, "And that's the way it is with stress. If we carry our burdens all the time, sooner or later, as the burden becomes increasingly heavy, we won't be able to carry on."

"As with the glass of water, you have to put down stress for a while and rest before holding it again. When we're refreshed, we can carry on with the burden—holding stress longer and better each time practiced. So, as early in the evening as you can, put all your burdens down. Don't carry them through the evening and into the night. Pick them up tomorrow."

Although stress is part of life, and certainly part of life when your child is seriously ill, it does not have to rule your life. Stress can be controlled and its negative effects diminished if not completely resolved. Common advice to better manage stress and care for yourself includes incorporating physical activity, relaxation techniques, meditation, yoga, or tai chi into your life.

Talking to friends and family decreases stress. As one mother said, "When I talk to others, I may learn something that will help my daughter. Even if I don't, I know that I am less alone. Talking is a good thing." Some parents will seek professional counseling to manage stress. The benefits of managing stress are better sleep, weight control, fewer bouts of sickness and faster healing, decrease in chronic aches and pain, improved mood, and better relationships with family and friends.

### How to Manage Stress

- Plan your time. Think ahead about how you are going to use your time and what you want to get done. Sometimes writing a to-do list helps you to decide what is most important. Be realistic about how much you can do.
- Prepare yourself. If you know something is coming up, picture the event in your mind. Stay positive. Have a backup plan.
- Relax with deep breathing or progressive muscle relaxation. Helpguide.org offers step-by-step instructions on their Relaxation Techniques for Stress Relief page (www.helpguide.org/mental/ stress_relief_meditation_yoga_relaxation.htm) (see Appendix).
- Increase your physical activity. Aim for 2½ hours each week of moderate aerobic activity, like fast walking or biking. Do strengthening activities, such as sit-ups or lifting weights, at least twice a week.
- Eat healthy. Give your body plenty of fruits and vegetables, and drink plenty of water.
- Drink alcohol only in moderation. This means no more than one drink per day for women or two drinks per day for men. Do not manage stress with alcohol, drugs, or tobacco.
- Declutter. Pick one area to tackle, such as your junk drawer, the piles of clothes in the bedroom, or the hall closet. Take a good look at what you have accumulated and then start by clearing out any items you do not use. If they are in good condition, consider donating them to an appropriate charity. Sort through what is left and be sure it is in the best place to be used and useful. If it is not, move it. Consider simplifying your schedule, too.

## Caregiving and Caring for Self

The Rosalynn Carter Institute for Caregivers, founded by former first lady Rosalynn Carter, offers a roadmap for those who find themselves unprepared to face the serious illness of a loved one. That is just about anyone facing the serious illness of an adult child (Carter & Golant, 1994).

- First, educate yourself. With your child's permission, this may be accomplished by asking questions of their healthcare provider. Other information can be obtained from reading and searching online or at the library. Information about the specific disease or illness is helpful. This gives you background information and information about what to expect. The Web site Patients Like Me (www.patientslikeme.com) is designed to put patients first. Its motto "You are not alone" will be comforting to many.

- Second, because much is outside of your control when it comes to the illness, try to control what you can. This will help you cope. This may be time for yourself that includes gardening, reading, or exercise—whatever you enjoy.

- Peer support groups can be a source of information and help. Often they also provide information about community resources, create networking connections, and give you an outlet to vent, including laughing, crying, and complaining. Some ways to find a support group include asking your or your child's healthcare provider, looking in the phone book or online, checking with your county health department, and contacting local religious or service organizations or government hotlines.

- Everyone needs support, but support groups are not for everyone. If you are a person who does not like to join groups, find someone to talk to. This one-on-one interaction will provide you support and some of the other benefits mentioned previously.

- For parents of seriously ill adult children, support groups are not common. You may identify support online through Ill Adult Children (www.illadultchildren.com).
- It is OK to back away if you cannot do something that is asked. It is OK to say no. Offer alternatives if any are available, but remember it is OK to say no.

 Other helpful strategies include

- Acknowledge your limitations.
- Focus on your loved one's strengths.
- Learn relaxation techniques.
- Take care of your health.
- Maintain a life outside of your parenting role.
- Keep a daily "burnout" log that records stressful events.
- Insist on private time, and build a caregiving team so you and your child are not alone.
- Rely on your sense of humor.
- Appreciate the benefits of leisure time.
- Help your child find a support group.
- Seek professional help.
- Appreciate your own efforts.
- Seek spiritual renewal.

## Julie's Story

Julie says, "I know that I have to take care of myself so that I can be with Jen physically and emotionally." For this she hangs on to the dualities of anger and support. "My anger propels me in a positive way. It keeps me going. I walk four or five times a week, take my medications as prescribed, and eat healthily." At the same time, she recognizes the role that others around her play. "Through activities, volunteering, and family, I have tremendous support. They are unbelievable."

She never attended or searched out a support group. Julie didn't know if one that would be appropriate even existed in her area. Why didn't she look? "I never pursued a support group since you tend to live in denial for so long or are so tired of talking about it. I guess going to a support group makes you relive it over again, which is tough," she reflects.

Julie uses e-mail communication with family and friends. These shared updates are not as time consuming or emotionally wringing as a separate conversation with everyone.

For Julie, taking care of herself also includes emotional care. In the past, she has used a therapist to help her with difficult times and the techniques she learned are helpful at this time. She has learned to be direct and confront a problem. She models this directness for her family members. "We do not take on other people's problems. By this I mean we do not allow undermining or talking against someone, against someone who is not present. We try to say what we mean and stay positive. It is not easy but the effort is worth it."

Julie has had to reassure little Lucas that she will always be there for him. And with true love, Lucas has also reassured her. "I will always be there for you, too, Grandma," he whispered back to her.

Through all of this, Julie says, "I need Jen as much as she needs me. We have always been close, but helping her gives me a purpose in a situation which I cannot control. It keeps the feelings of helplessness away."

# Conclusion

Caregiving and illness are stressful occurrences. Learning to care for yourself physically, emotionally, and spiritually will keep you in the best shape to manage negative effects. This has the added benefit of positively affecting your adult child because you are able to provide needed help so that he may focus better on his treatment.

# References

Carter, R., & Golant, S.K. (1994). *Helping yourself help others.* New York, NY: Random House.

Grinyer, A. (2006). Caring for a young adult with cancer: The impact on mothers' health. *Health and Social Care in the Community, 14,* 311–318. doi:10.1111/j.1365-2524.2006.00622.x

Mayo Clinic. (2011a, February 10). Broken heart syndrome. Retrieved from http://www.mayoclinic.com/health/broken-heart-syndrome/DS01135

Mayo Clinic. (2011b, March 19). Stress management. Retrieved from http://www.mayoclinic.com/health/stress-management/MY00435

Mitnick, S., Leffler, C., & Hood, V.L. (2010). Family caregivers, patients and physicians: Ethical guidance to optimize relationships. *Journal of General Internal Medicine, 25,* 255–260. doi:10.1007/s11606-009-1206-3

Pinchot, L.J. (2011). *Help wanted: Caregiver.* Pittsburgh, PA: Hygeia Media.

Raveis, V.H., Pretter, S., & Carrero, M. (2010). "It should have been happening to me": The psychosocial issues older caregiving mothers experience. *Journal of Family Social Work, 13,* 131–148. doi:10.1080/10522150903503002

**By the Way...**

- Take care of yourself. Start today with a hot shower or bath and talking to a trusted friend.
- Deep breathing, progressive muscle relaxation, meditation, yoga, and tai chi all help decrease and manage stress. For guidance, consult an instructor, written resources, or an online program.
- Open, honest communication with your child and others you are close to will decrease stress and allow better care and relationships.
- Keep a journal Using a pretty book to write down positive and negative feelings, to-do lists, and things that must be remembered will increase clarity and control. The pretty book makes it easier to write in and to read.
- Seek professional counseling if you need to discuss things with someone other than your friends and family.
- Recognize and accept all your emotions and feelings as normal. You cannot control how you feel, only your actions.
- As much as you can, plan your time, recognizing that the unexpected will happen.
- Move. Aim for 2½ hours of physical activity each week or 20 minutes each day.
- Eat and drink healthily.
- Declutter one area of your life that you control.
- Educate yourself about your child's medical condition and care. In doing this, follow the limits set by your adult child.
- Use face-to-face or online support groups if they fit your needs.
- Find peer support either in a group or with an individual. The Web site Ill Adult Children (www.illadultchildren.com) may help.
- Know that you can say no.

# CHAPTER 9

# THE NEED FOR HELP:
# Understanding the Healthcare System

*In preparing for battle, I have found that planning is essential, but plans are useless.*

—Dwight Eisenhower

## Helen's Story

"Shelly was never a 'normal' child. She is bipolar with weight extreme highs and lows. She is selfish and she always was . . . she always had to have the best of everything. Family counseling when she was younger did little to stop her running away, skipping school, smoking, or drinking," Shelly's mother, Helen, recalls. Helen had to deal with all of this before Shelly was diagnosed with AIDS at the age of 35. Now she is 41 years old and a recent MRI of the brain showed AIDS dementia.

Although Shelly was married and living in Pennsylvania, she met someone online who lived in New York. She left her husband and moved to New York. She seemed happy. "I sort of monitor this, her happiness and stability, by her weight, and her weight had been steady at about 165 pounds," explains Helen. "She was back in school for medical transcription when later that year her weight dropped to 118 pounds. She stopped taking her medications and she flunked out of school."

Helen is Shelly's surrogate for healthcare decisions and went to New York at this crisis. When she arrived, Shelly was incapable of making her own decisions. Her weight was 88 pounds and the physician asked for a do-not-resuscitate (DNR) order. Helen refused and moved Shelly back to Pennsylvania. For the past three months, this decision to move Shelly back home has put them on a roller coaster ride with healthcare benefits and the healthcare system. It seems that because she was not considered a resident of Pennsylvania, the coverage was different. In New York, Medicaid and Social Security covered the majority of health-related expenses. For example, Shelly's AIDS medications cost $2,000 per month.

Helen goes on, "Shelly's short-term memory is for crap. I go to her apartment twice a day to check that she is taking her medications correctly. Her long-term memory is no prize either. She sometimes confuses what she has seen in the movies with her life. It is really, really difficult."

"I am fighting for her care all the time. Most recently it is with the local Office on Aging, which represents extended care facilities. The facility where Shelly was admitted for rehabilitation, exercises and stuff, determined that she could be discharged from this nursing home and go live at the homeless shelter. What kind of a plan is that?" Helen asks. "They did not notify me before discharging her, and I only found out when I went to visit her the next day. Besides, she has her own apartment. If they would have asked me, I would have told them that."

"I'm not a quitter and I don't take 'no' for an answer," Helen says of her tenacity and developing advocacy skills.

"Unfortunately, I am always fighting with Shelly, too," says Helen. "I know she resents me helping her or telling her what to do, but what choice do I have? I love her, and I want her to be safe. I worry that she will leave her apartment and not turn off the lights or not turn off the stove."

"My husband is Shelly's stepfather, but he would do just about anything for her. The problem is he's germaphobic, at least that's what I call it. Ever since her AIDS diagnosis he will not touch her, and that hurts her. He can't help it."

Shelly did divorce her husband and then marry the man she ran away to New York to be with, but he could not handle her illness. Now he wants to reconcile, but she is not the same woman he married. They remain separated. He is not helping her at this time.

## The Healthcare System

In order for patients and their families to obtain what they need from the healthcare system, they must first understand the basics of that system. Some fundamental information can help you understand the system. These fundamentals include the who, what, and where of health care.

### Who

The healthcare team is who provides health care. When referring to the healthcare team, that usually means the physician, nurse, nurse assistant or aide, social worker, and chaplain. These people form the core of the healthcare team and will obtain assistance from others to meet special needs such as the pharmacist, dietitian, physical therapist, occupational therapist, and speech therapist. Here's what they do.

- Physicians or doctors diagnose and treat medical problems. Generally considered team leaders, doctors give orders to other team members, have completed the required schooling, and have successfully passed all licensing tests to practice medicine. Physicians are further categorized by specialty and type of practice.

  – *Primary care physicians* or *family physicians* are the health professionals individuals initially see when ill or for periodic health checks; these physicians coordinate the care when patients have multiple health concerns and multiple physicians involved in their care.

  – *Resident physicians* are completing training after medical school in an area of specialty.

  – *Physician assistants* are not doctors but work under the direction of a supervising physician performing tasks that are delegated to them.

  – *Hospitalist* is a new specialty. These physicians work at usually just one hospital and see patients throughout their hospital stay. Communication with the primary care physicians or family physicians is maintained, but the hospitalist cares for the patient during hospitalization.

- Nurses assess and assist patients and families in adapting to life circumstances, particularly alterations caused by medical problems. A variety of nursing staff may be involved in care. What all nurses have in common is that they have completed a particular education program and successfully passed a licensing test. That being said, they may still vary by the amount of education and the type of licensure. Advanced practice nurses have completed graduate education with either a master's degree or a doctorate degree. These nurses work with physicians but are the most independent, often seeing patients without a physician but always having access to a physician or supervising physician.

- *Nurse assistants or aides* are unlicensed staff members who assist with basic patient care such as giving baths and checking vital signs. Preparation usually consists of completing a training course.

- *Social workers* are professional members of the team whose expertise is linking the patient with community resources. Some social workers also provide counseling.

- *Chaplains* provide spiritual care. Although usually associated with a particular religion and driven by their own faith beliefs, their role is not to convert or proselytize but to support the spiritual needs of patients.

- *Pharmacists* are educated and licensed to prepare and dispense drugs and associated educational information.

- *Dietitians* supervise the preparation and service of food, develop modified diets, and educate individuals and groups on good nutritional habits and lifestyles.

- *Therapists* are healthcare team members who are skilled in giving therapy, usually in a specific healthcare field. Examples include speech therapists, physical therapists, and respiratory therapists.

Other professionals may be less visible at the bedside but can help you understand the healthcare system or troubleshoot problems that arise.

- Although two different positions, *patient representatives* or *ombudsmen* are both experts at solving problems and resolving complaints. Both act as advocates, verify complaints, and work for their resolution. These professionals are experienced in a wide range of issues from financial to care delivery to ethical problems.

- *Patient navigator* is a newer role that is designated to someone who can explain and support the care that is planned. They are usually responsible for providing education and support to the patient and family along with ensuring that nothing is missed.

These core roles and responsibilities can be further specialized. For example, an orthopedic surgeon is a physician who operates only on bones; an oncology nurse cares for patients with cancer; a hospice nursing assistant works only with patients at the end of life; a pediatric social worker works only with children and their families; and a chaplain can be a certified hospital chaplain. These examples are a few of the numerous specialized roles. With each introduction, you should ask what the person's role is in your child's care. If you do not understand what they tell you, ask them to explain.

In an academic center, such as a university hospital, you may also have contact with people on the healthcare team who have not completed their education or specialization. They may be working temporarily in an area to gain experience or to specialize. You do not need to fear these people or the care they give. Hospital programs provide supervision with a clear hierarchy or chain of command. Students and residents have instructors and supervisors instructing them and watching. Sometimes they may be a phone call away, but never farther than that.

## What and Where

The *what* and *where* of health care go hand-in-hand. That is, the type of care needed will determine where someone will go, and where someone goes will depend on what kind of care is needed. The level of care determines the appropriate facility.

One way to distinguish the kinds of care is based on acuity. *Acuity* refers to the severity of an illness with the more acute illnesses requiring hospitalization. The more acute, or higher acuity, usually means a sicker patient. As medical conditions are cured or controlled, care may switch to either outpatient settings, such as clinics and physician offices, or more long-term and less acute inpatient settings, such as extended-care facilities or rehabilitation centers. The healthcare team strives to give the right care at the right time in the right place to the right patient.

# Help From the Healthcare Team: Care Coordination Models

With a serious illness, the patient, family and loved ones, and all members of the healthcare team must communicate with one another. Improvements are being made in how care is delivered in these most complex of situations. In general, this is referred to as care coordination and may occur within a setting such as a hospital or between settings such as a clinic and home care. A hallmark of these models is collaboration of all who are involved with care. Strategies employed to improve care coordination generally encompass new technology and improve upon existing technology such as electronic medical records, automated cell phone text messaging, automated electronic monthly educational messages, and telephone reminders for appointments and testing. One characteristic shared by many—if not all—care coordination models is patient engagement: involving the patients and their support system in improving their healthcare and disease management. Some brief descriptions are given here.

- *Chronic care or medical home model* is designed as a team-based approach with the primary care physician as the leader. Longer scheduled visits allow thorough chronic disease management and preventive care to help patient confidence and self-management skills. This model attempts to decrease unnecessary hospitalizations and emergency department visits while improving access to care for the patient.

- *Case management models* usually feature a nurse as the primary point of contact within the healthcare team. This nurse provides primary care, coordination, and support services to patients, education about self-care, and referrals to community programs and services.

- *Disease management programs* span the continuum of care, for example, a program for people with congestive heart failure that refocuses sites where care is delivered. The goal is to decrease emergency department visits and increase the focus on rehabilitation and education.

- *Patient navigator model* may include a nurse, social worker, or another healthcare professional to help direct care across different settings, institutions, and disease trajectories. This is becoming common with cancer care from diagnostic testing through treatment and survival or end-of-life care.

- *Palliative care model* benefits patients with life-threatening illness who are identified earlier than the end of life. The goal is to enhance communication regarding care goals and treatment burdens to ensure these are respected as early in the disease trajectory as possible. This model of care supports both curative and end-of-life therapies. Attention to pain and symptom management, clear communication, and goals of care are hallmarks.

- *Hospice care* is also palliative care but is specific for end-of-life care, usually for patients with a six-month life expectancy and no curative treatment intents. This is often covered by insurance and provides help to care for the dying.

The key elements of successful care transitions include choosing the best next care setting when needed; arranging appropriate and needed services; receiving verbal, written, and electronic patient and family education and support; and maintaining clear communication among team members and settings that includes the course of care, key test results, the current care plan for treatment, current medication lists, and what follow-up care and appointments are needed.

Knowing as much as possible about the care your adult child received or is receiving and the healthcare professional who is giving the care may improve the outcome. With your child's permission, it will also enable you to better help your child. Advocacy is one way to ensure that quality care is delivered appropriately and that needs are met.

# Advocacy

First published in 1973 by the American Hospital Association (AHA, 2003), the Patient's Bill of Rights emphasized the responsibilities of hospitals and patients and the need to communicate and collaborate for the best care. It outlined the scope for both the patient and the hospital, which includes the patient's right to care that is respectful and appropriate. This document has subsequently been replaced by AHA with a more readable version for patients and families, *What to Expect During Your Hospital Stay*. This brochure is an example of healthcare advocacy and outlines basic care that all healthcare consumers should expect during a hospital stay, including (AHA, 2003)

• High-quality hospital care
• A clean and safe environment
• Involvement in your care
• Protection of your privacy
• Help when leaving the hospital
• Help with your billing claims.

   Advocacy is speaking up, that is, the pleading or representation for a desired goal or interest group. It encompasses speaking up for your own care or the care of your loved one. In Helen's story, her advocacy skills developed out of necessity. She was determined to understand the system and secure for her daughter the help she needed. Advocacy is not just speaking up to be heard but to accomplish something. This may be care for an individual, help with a bill, or the selection of an appropriate care facility. Countless groups would be considered advocacy groups and range from grassroots organizations to professional societies.

   In his 2012 book, *The Best Care Possible*, Dr. Ira Byock, director of Palliative Medicine at Dartmouth-Hitchcock Medical Center in New Hampshire, developed his own list of reasonable expectations when seriously ill patients and their families are interacting with the healthcare team and system (p. 244):

- To have one's pain and other physical symptoms regularly assessed and competently treated.
- To have adequate information about one's condition and treatments, in clear and simple terms.
- To have care coordinated between visits and among physicians and health programs involved in one's care.
- To have crises prevented when possible and have clear plans for managing emergencies in place.
- To have enough nurses and aides on staff in hospitals and nursing homes to provide safe and high-quality care.
- To have one's family supported in giving care, in their own strain, and, eventually, in grief.

## Health Insurance Portability and Accountability Act

Another significant advocacy effort on behalf of patients is the Health Insurance Portability and Accountability Act (HIPAA) of 1996 (U.S. Department of Health and Human Services, n.d.). This federal law, issued by the U.S. Department of Health and Human Services, legally protects the privacy of patient information. A major goal of this law is to ensure that individuals' health information is properly protected from unauthorized review and use while allowing the flow of health information needed to provide and promote high-quality health care and to protect the public's health and well-being. It strikes a balance that permits important uses of information while protecting the privacy of people who seek care. Individually identifiable health information held or transmitted by a covered entity or its business associate, in any form or media, whether electronic, paper, or oral, is protected. This information is known as *protected health information.*

Because the privacy of adult health information is protected, healthcare providers have a legal and ethical obligation to protect patient confidentiality. HIPAA gives adults control over the release of health information and is not designed to be difficult or obstructive. It is also not intended to be disrespectful of the parent but rather is intended to be respectful of your adult child who is the patient or recipient of care.

Healthcare providers are very careful about releasing information about the patient's condition to anyone other than the patient. They are allowed to give information only with the patient's permission and only to those whom the patient identifies as allowed to receive information about his condition. With your child's consent you may be added to the list of those who are allowed to receive information. If you have your child's permission to obtain information, you may ask them about any passwords in use. There are some questions that have been prepared by the Agency for Healthcare Research and Quality (AHRQ) that will guide you and keep you on track when gathering information to help your child make decisions. If your child does not give consent for you to receive healthcare information, healthcare providers have no choice but to refuse to release information to you.

**The 10 Questions You Should Ask Your Healthcare Provider**

Never be afraid or intimidated about asking a question. A simple question can make a big difference, letting you take better care of yourself or even saving your life or that of your loved one. The questions below can get you started.

1. What is the test for?
2. How many times have you done this procedure?
3. When will I get the results?
4. Why do I need this treatment?
5. Are there any alternatives?
6. What are the possible complications?
7. Which hospital is best for my needs?
8. How do you spell the name of that drug?
9. Are there any side effects?
10. Will this medicine interact with medicines that I'm already taking?

*Note.* From "Questions Are the Answer: Better Communication. Better Care," by the Agency for Healthcare Research and Quality, n.d. Retrieved from http://www.ahrq.gov/questions.

# Quality Care

We want the best care for ourselves and for our children. Donald Berwick (2004), in his book *Escape Fire: Designs for the Future of Health Care*, recounts what quality care is for Kevin, a 15-year-old with short gut syndrome who has had surgery nine times in 13 years to replace his feeding tube—"three things about the care he received that especially pleased him—what he would call 'quality'—and three things he identified as 'defects'" (pp. 6–7).

Care is best when:

• They tell you what's going on right away.

- You get the same answer from everyone.
- They don't make you scared.
  Care is worst when:
- They keep you waiting.
- They don't listen to what you say, even when sometimes you know better.
- They do everything twice instead of once.

Just like Kevin, everyone wants quality care. Quality health care can be defined in a number of ways. How quality is determined and rated is complex, and finding this information is not always easy.

According to AHRQ Director Dr. Carolyn Clancy (2008), doing your homework will help ensure you get good quality care.

Private groups, such as the Department of Health Care Policy at Harvard Medical School (www.hcp.med.harvard. edu), produce hospital report cards. These hospital "grades" are based on different measures, which should be clearly stated. For example, some grade hospitals on what doctors think of them, whether the hospital uses computers to order drugs, and how well patients recover from different kinds of surgeries. These report cards are voluntary, and hospitals are not required to participate in them. This could mean that no data may be available about a specific hospital. Another problem is that some organizations often use data that are several years old.

You can also find out more about a specific hospital's overall quality of care and how it compares with other hospitals in your area. The U.S. Department of Health and Human Services has a useful source of information on hospital quality. The

Hospital Compare Web site (www.hospitalcompare.hhs.gov) provides information about how well hospitals care for adult patients with certain conditions. The majority of hospitals—about 90%—report their quality data. Hospital Compare offers information such as

• How often a hospital gives the right treatments for certain conditions, such as heart attacks, heart failure, and pneumonia, or procedures, such as preventing surgical infections

• Typical results of care or treatment for certain conditions or procedures

• How much Medicare paid hospitals for certain conditions and procedures

• Patients' perception about the care they received during a recent hospital stay. Their experiences are an important part of good quality care. Feedback from patients to more than two dozen questions is currently available. Information from most of the nation's hospitals should soon be available on the Hospital Compare Web site.

The largest agency that accredits hospitals in the United States is the Joint Commission. This national, nonprofit organization's Web site, Quality Check (www.qualitycheck.org), offers a searchable database of information for any hospital in the United States. This site can tell you whether a hospital is accredited and will identify hospitals that have not met quality standards.

Measuring hospital quality isn't a perfect science, but information is available to help you make educated decisions. Those are the best decisions for peace of mind and for health.

## Evidence-Based Medicine

What is *evidence-based medicine*? It is a term that you see a lot when determining quality care and the best care, but what does it mean? It refers to the amount or level of research studies available that support a given treatment. Most often this is in the literature for healthcare professionals. True and surprising is the fact that many healthcare decisions are made without strong evidence on their effectiveness and lack of harm. To be useful, information should be scientifically valid, trustworthy, and understandable for patients who wish to work constructively with their clinicians to make the best medical decisions for themselves (ECRI Institute, n.d.).

## The Cochrane Collaboration

An easily accessible body of evidence for health care is the Cochrane Collaboration. The main purpose of the Cochrane Collaboration is to develop systematic reviews of the strongest evidence available about healthcare interventions. Consumers and health practitioners can then work together to make the best possible decisions about health care. The reviews are published electronically within the Cochrane Library (www.cochrane .org) and are freely accessible in shortened versions. The Collaboration is a nonprofit organization based in the United Kingdom. To carry out its mission of producing systematic reviews, a central administration supports disease- and health condition–based groups (Cochrane Review Groups) who work with authors and editors to develop systematic reviews. The review groups are spread across the world, generally based at universities and teaching hospitals. The main activity of the Collaboration is the preparation of Cochrane reviews that are published electronically in successive issues of the Cochrane Library.

## Clinical Trials

The best evidence in health care is obtained from clinical trials. These are not guinea pig experiments but carefully developed studies that are reviewed by leaders in the field. If a clinical trial is considered for treatment, you can be assured that the treatment has been proved to be as good as the standard of care with the potential of offering something better before it is offered to human study participants. Much measuring and reporting is associated with participating in a clinical trial. Some patients may find this bothersome, but it is the best way to gather evidence or data.

In 2002, the ECRI Institute, an independent, nonprofit organization that researches the best approaches to improving the safety, quality, and cost-effectiveness of patient care, published the booklet *Should I Enter a Clinical Trial: A Guide for Adults With a Serious or Life-Threatening Illness.* Seriously ill patients often and increasingly seek cutting-edge treatments that are still being tested in clinical trials and are not yet part of routine or standard care in the healthcare system. Whether to enter a clinical trial and which trial to enter are important issues (ECRI Institute, 2002).

# Helen's Story

Helen has two children, Shelly and her younger brother. They have never been close, and her son does not understand any of Shelly's needs. He interprets it all as attention-seeking. "Unfortunately each child thinks I love the other one more," she explains.

Support is important for Helen, and she actively seeks it from her husband, mother-in-law, family, and girlfriends.

She talks about her husband's cousin, Linda, whose adult son developed encephalitis from a mosquito bite as a child. "I watched her care for him over the years. His mental capacity is that of about a six-year-old, and he has the behavior problems that accompany it. I always felt sorry for her. Now I think, 'If she can do it, so can I.'

"I am also very organized and so is Shelly. I guess she gets that from me. At least I did something right," she says thoughtfully.

"Shelly cannot or does not accept her physical and mental changes. Her old friends have stopped calling her, and some have even changed their phone numbers to discontinue contact with her. It is hard for a mother to watch the hurt that happens, but I do see how she is different. I know that she can be persistent to the point of harassing."

As for Helen: how hard is Shelly on her? "I love her," she replies simply. She continues to advocate and interact with the healthcare team and healthcare system on Shelly's behalf.

# Conclusion

This chapter provided an understanding of the healthcare system. With your child's permission, your understanding should include who is caring for your child, what is being done for treatment, and how to ask about the quality of care. The art and science of health care is the continual pursuit of the best care.

# References

American Hospital Association. (2003). *The patient care partnership: Understanding expectations, rights, and responsibilities.* Retrieved from http://www.aha.org/content/00-10/pcp_english_030730.pdf

Berwick, D.M. (2004). *Escape fire: Designs for the future of health care.* San Francisco, CA: Jossey-Bass.

Byock, I. (2012). *The best care possible: A physician's quest to transform care through the end of life.* New York, NY: Avery.

Clancy, C.M. (2008, June 17). Do your homework before you choose a hospital. Retrieved from http://www.ahrq.gov/consumer/cc/cc061708.htm

ECRI Institute. (n.d.). Our vision for a national patient library. Retrieved from https://www.ecri.org/Patients/References/Pages/ECRI_Institute_Vision_for_a_National_Patient_Library.aspx

ECRI Institute. (2002). Should I enter a clinical trial? A patient reference guide for adults with a serious or life-threatening illness. Retrieved from https://www.ecri.org/Patients/References/Pages/Clinical_Trials_Patient_Reference_Guide.aspx

U.S. Department of Health and Human Services. (n.d.). Summary of the HIPAA Privacy Rule. Retrieved from http://www.hhs.gov/ocr/privacy/hipaa/understanding/summary/index.html

**By the Way...**

- If your child has given permission for you to receive health information from the healthcare team, be sure that it is in writing and that you know any passwords or identifiers.
- With each introduction to new members of the healthcare team, ask what their role is in your child's care. If you do not understand what they tell you, ask them to explain.
- Have all your questions answered. If one professional does not know, ask him to direct you to someone else on the healthcare team who may have the answers.
- Your questions about quality care may also be answered through independent research online with agencies such as the Joint Commission, the Agency for Healthcare Research and Quality, and Hospital Compare.
- There is more information about being an engaged patient available online. Some resources include
  - e-Patient Dave, a Voice of Patient Engagement (http://epatientdave.com)
  - The Leapfrog Group (http://leapfroggroup.org)
  - Health Grades (www.healthgrades.com)
- Strategies for successful advocacy with healthcare team members on behalf of your child (Byock, 2012):
  - Be polite, pleasant, and persistent.
  - Learn the names of staff and befriend them if possible.
  - Tell staff about your child so they begin to know him as a person. Bringing pictures into the room may help with this.
  - Say thank you.
  - If the care that is given is not meeting the needs of your child, stand your ground politely. Your child's needs are more important than the staff's feelings.
- Information is power. To be informed, it is important to know what questions to ask. Keep The 10 Questions You Should Ask Your Healthcare Provider from this chapter handy for conversations with healthcare providers.
- Reliable online information for various diseases and medical conditions include WebMD (www.webmd.com), the Mayo Clinic (www.mayoclinic.org), and the Cleveland Clinic (http://my.clevelandclinic.org), to name just three of many.

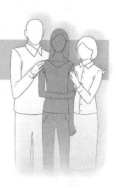

# CHAPTER 10

# WANTING TO KNOW BUT AFRAID TO ASK:
# Prognosis

*Fear is forward. No one is afraid of yesterday.*

—Renata Adler

## Bonnie's Story

Bonnie is in her late 70s. Her gray wristband proclaims "age well, live strong" but her looks and conversation would easily allow you to mistake her for a much younger woman. A volunteer healthcare advocate for seniors, she has also been a medical technologist and administrator for a nonprofit organization. While her three daughters were growing up, the family lived in different locations in South America and the United States, moving to follow her husband's job.

She talked about two of her daughters and their struggles with serious illness as adults. Mary, a beautiful young woman, had been injured in a motor vehicle accident when she was 18 years old. Her injuries were both physical and psychological. After rehabilitation and recovery, Mary still required some assistance to care for herself and to walk. Determined to live independently, she met and married a man who was neglectful and abusive. Eventually he kicked her out of the home, and she moved back with her parents. While living with her parents, Mary was diagnosed with lung cancer. Bonnie didn't think Mary had ever smoked, but she had lived with chain-smokers the past seven years. She died at the age of 34.

About 20 years later, Bonnie's daughter Kelly suffered a series of small but debilitating strokes. She was 50 years old. Diabetes and obesity were known risk factors, but nothing prepares you for the call that your child is in critical condition in the emergency department.

Flashbacks and flash-forwards immediately bombarded Bonnie when she heard the news. The experience with Mary had made it difficult to pull back, but Kelly was older and had a husband who was interested in caring for his wife and making decisions to support both of them.

"You always have to put the spouse's relationship first unless it is detrimental to your child's well-being," she had learned.

Another noticeable difference between her roles in the two daughters' illnesses was how she was perceived by the healthcare team. When her 18-year-old daughter was injured, although she was legally an adult, Bonnie was always consulted and kept informed. With Kelly, very few healthcare professionals acknowledged her. Any information that she received came from her daughter or her daughter's husband. Although her interest was no less intense than it was earlier, her access to information was achingly limited.

## Prognosis

What will happen next? What can be expected? *Prognosis* is the prediction of the course and end of a disease and the estimate of chance for recovery. This chapter explores issues of prognosis and related topics. First it will look at the possible outcomes of a serious illness, including survivorship, resiliency, post-traumatic stress disorder (PTSD), and even death; it then moves to advance care planning, as well as the associated difficult discussions and decisions. Yes, much more than just emotions can affect prognosis.

It is notoriously hard to predict medical outcomes accurately. No one has a crystal ball that works. Observation and research have shown that physicians are not particularly good or accurate at predicting the outcome of an illness. This is especially true when trying to predict how much longer a person will live. Physicians are inaccurate in their prognoses for terminally ill patients and usually overly optimistic (Christakis & Lamont, 2000; Yourman, Lee, Schonberg, Widera, & Smith, 2012).

Often, prognosis encompasses answers to the feared questions—the scary ones. Prognosis is often colored by its surroundings. What treatments have been tried? What is the age of the child? What other medical conditions are present? The illness itself also determines the prognosis: What is the stage of disease? Is it curable? Will there be disability or death? Is it acute or chronic or sudden?

## Outcomes of a Serious Illness

There are as many variations of the outcomes of a serious illness as there are the stories of the people so affected. Simplistically, the outcomes of a serious illness could be a full recovery, control of a chronic condition, or death.

*Full recovery* describes Caroline after completing surgery and radiation treatments for a very small, early breast cancer. She was cancer free.

Minnie has learned to *control* her dangerously high blood pressure. This was through treatment and rehabilitation following a stroke, after which she had to learn to walk again. It was difficult, and the threat of further problems is always present. PTSD and resilience are two possible outcomes of serious illness, treatment, and survivorship.

Death can also be an outcome of a serious illness. Gloria's son developed a rare, aggressive, and ultimately fatal cancer. Despite surgery and chemotherapy, about two years after the diagnosis was made, her 30-year-old son was receiving hospice care. Later she would say, "No one should have to call in hospice professionals to help care for your child." He had moved back home with her, and she was the primary caregiver until his death. With the help of a hospice organization, who had someone ready to help her 24/7, she got a hospital bed in the living room, made his favorite foods, and later offered sips of juice and flavored ice. The hospice staff ensured that she knew how to give the medications, and when his pain medications would seem to not be working, adjustments in the medications were made. During that time and afterward, she recalls, "I pulled myself together again each and every day." Three months later he died in his childhood home with his mother caring for him. Death is a very real possibility with a serious illness, but not for everyone.

## Survivorship

There is no agreement on the definition of a survivor. It is increasingly common, when talking about surviving cancer, to describe survival beginning at the time of diagnosis. Dr. Anne Katz, clinical nurse specialist, adjunct professor at the University of Manitoba, and editor of the *Oncology Nursing Forum*, describes the history of the term and the current thinking in her book, *After You Ring the Bell . . . Ten Challenges for the Cancer Survivor* (2012). It is fair to say that survivors are diverse. This group includes those just diagnosed, those in active treatment, those in rehabilitation, those who have successfully completed treatment, and all those in between.

Agreement on who is a survivor in other diseases also carries some ambiguity. It may be that survivorship is completing a recommended course of treatment for a life-threatening illness; the disease may be cured or controlled. It may be helpful to conceptualize survivorship along a continuum with early and later phases of survivorship. This survivorship trajectory highlights that you do not just "get over" a serious illness.

When active treatment ends, there is no doubt it is a cause for celebration. But the end of treatment or therapy also causes trepidation. It implies responsibility for future wellness. Unlike Minnie, who after her stroke recovery said she just wanted to forget all about it, the course and treatment of a serious illness must be remembered. It does not have to be constantly remembered, but it must be recorded. It can affect the rest of one's life. To be most proactive and successful, a survivorship care plan checklist is recommended.

A survivorship care plan checklist includes

- A treatment summary with the type and stage of disease, date diagnosed, and types of treatment received, including surgical procedures, names of drugs, radiation doses, complications experienced, including side effects, hospitalizations, and transfusions, other treatments, and rehabilitation measures.
- A follow-up healthcare plan starting with a description of state of health at the end of treatment, future schedule of visits (when, where, and with whom), tests that will be done, possible long-term effects that might occur, and symptoms to watch for that might signal a recurrence.
- A wellness plan covering important lifelong health habits and screening tests for other diseases that may or may not be related to the individual's health history.

## Post-Traumatic Stress Disorder

As previously mentioned, Caroline had an early-stage breast cancer. Her cancer was diagnosed by a routine screening mammogram. Treatment with surgery and radiation therapy followed, and she successfully completed it. From her physicians' point of view, she was cured. Caroline was not so certain. The next time she had a routine screening test, a colonoscopy when she turned 50 years old, in her words, "I freaked out!" She remembered all too vividly how her last screening test, a mammogram, had turned out. The trauma of that mammogram and subsequent diagnosis of breast cancer caused Caroline to be unreasonably fearful of all routine cancer screening tests. Caroline's response is an example of post-traumatic stress disorder, or PTSD.

PTSD was first applied to patients with cancer in the 1990s. By definition it is the development of characteristic symptoms following exposure to an extremely traumatic stressor. The diagnosis encompasses severe and disabling anxiety and phobic reactions following a traumatic experience. Any serious illness and its subsequent treatment can be traumatic.

Much of the research about PTSD and serious illness comes from studies about cancer survivors. According to Nancy Jo Bush, a cancer survivor and professor at the University of California, Los Angeles, "The fight against cancer is unknown, frightening, and a threat to self-integrity. Until the last decade, what has not been known is that some patients do not psychologically recover from the diagnosis, treatments, and unpredictable future as readily as others" (Bush, 2010, p. E334). One of the traumatic hallmarks of the cancer experience is that multiple crises and stressors occur with this disease and treatment. It is not just one bomb exploding but several—the diagnosis, the treatments and side effects, the possibility of recurrence, and recurrence are examples of some stressors.

As one breast cancer survivor quipped, "My telomeres must be really short by now," referring to the ends of her chromosomes that act to protect our genetic material during cell division. Telomeres are thought to shorten with age, maybe with stress, and eventually when they are too short, cell death occurs. After a life of adapting to stress, including a sister with a poorly controlled seizure disorder, the death of an infant son, and her mother's breast cancer diagnosis followed by her own breast cancer diagnosis and treatment, her observation was, "I buffer every day of my life. I also learned to fight and adapt.

The breast cancer diagnosis was not my first call to fight for something important."

Perceived social support has been shown to be protective against PTSD. Particularly important for those with PTSD is the ability to form and maintain trusting and safe relationships with their caregivers. Other ways to prevent or relieve PTSD include

• A quiet, relaxing environment
• Relaxation techniques such as guided imagery
• Art and music therapy
• Professional counseling.

Interpersonal resources that promote positive coping and adaptation include resilience, hopefulness, optimism, self-efficacy, emotional intelligence, and spirituality. Fostering these will help your child, no matter the outcome of the illness.

In *My Stroke of Insight: A Brain Scientist's Personal Journey* (2008), Jill Bolte Taylor credits her mother as playing a big part as she recovered from a major stroke. Her mother knew what to do instinctively and that included holding her, lying beside her, and celebrating every little victory. Also valuable was that her mom, Gigi, remembered. Her mother would report back to Jill her progress because Jill's memory was severely damaged from the stroke. She could not remember from one moment to the next or from one day to the next. So, Gigi would remind her that last week she could only sit up in the chair for five minutes, and this week it is longer. These are examples of resilience. Resilience is a factor that enables some to overcome and transform profoundly traumatic life events.

## Resilience

Resilience is the ability to recover. The balance or equilibrium that is maintained through difficult circumstances is resilience. It is a composite of strength, flexibility, high self-esteem, hardiness, internal locus of control, autonomy, assertiveness, and humor. It allows meaning to come from an experience like cancer and movement toward recovery and healing. Resilience is not only innate but can be learned (Bush, 2010).

This may be what some people mean when they report that cancer or another serious illness has propelled them toward a spiritual search for meaning and self-transcendence. It may also be what others have expressed as an enriching experience, helping them to reprioritize what is important in their lives.

Resilience is important for the child, or anyone, who is seriously ill. It is also important for those who love and care for them. All of these lives are affected by a serious illness, and a new normal becomes reality.

In her 2009 book *Resilience: Reflections on the Burdens and Gifts of Facing Life's Adversities*, Elizabeth Edwards writes about this. In her lifetime she had experienced the death of a child, breast cancer, and her husband's well-publicized extramarital affair. As she said, "I have a lot of experience in getting up after I have been knocked down" (p. 27). ". . . I had to accept that the planet had taken a few turns and I could not turn it back. . . . Each time there was a new life, a new story. And the less time I spent trying to pretend that Wade was alive or that my life would be just as long or that my marriage would be as magical, the longer I clung to the hope that my old life might come back, the more I set myself up for unending discontent. . . . it took me some time just to get to acceptance, and in each case, that was only part of the way home" (pp. 31–32). Resiliency is not just bouncing back, or picking yourself up, or recovering; it is acknowledging the new reality and continuing on in a stable manner. It is regaining your balance with the changes that have occurred.

Edwards described resilience as recovering from the landmines that destroy the foundation of your life and then accepting a new reality. Illustrating strategies of what she did to help herself is enlightening, but she was not suggesting they are for everyone. Strategies for resilience that she practiced:

- Reaching out to online communities, griefnet.org and Web Healing, where she introduced Wade to those who did not know him. "But sharing Wade, making certain that to the extent I was able I parented his memory as well as a mother might, that made each day easier, which made the next day easier. I created a new place for him" (pp. 85–86).

- "The biggest step was having more children. Wade died in April of 1996. Emma Claire was born in April of 1998, and Jack was born in May of 2000. It was a conscious decision to have more children. What, John and I wondered in our new quiet house in Raleigh, will ever bring happiness back into the house in which Cate [the Edwards' daughter] will live? What brings us joy? The answer was clear: children. . . . We went to the doctor and I started a regimen of shots and medicines to increase the likelihood that we would have children. I was 48 when I had Emma Claire, and—with my AARP card in hand—I was 50 when I had Jack a month before Cate graduated from high school" (p. 102).

- "I wanted something that was mine. If I spoke publicly, I was asked about John. If I was asked to be on a board, it was because they had come to know me through John. I needed to be independent of him, maybe because he had been independent of me . . . I would open a furniture store" (p. 203). Individual ways to discover resilience take creativity. No one has ever lived a particular life before. Understanding a new normal takes time. It may involve

- Reflecting on what you have been through
- Identifying changes you might want to make in your life
- Recognizing what you have learned and what's changed about you
- Reevaluating personal relationships or professional goals
- Discovering new ways to find meaning and fulfillment.

As mentioned in Chapter 4, Patti's daughter, Kim, was diagnosed with ulcerative colitis while in college. Decisions had to be made about treatment and care but also about continuing her education. During the time she was actively bleeding, Kim wanted to stay and continue her studies at Ohio State University, a 2½-hour drive from home. Patti and her husband balked but had to assess the situation. Kim was living in a dorm on the seventh floor with a bathroom down the hall and a bunk bed she had to climb up to reach. But was it safe? Yes. Could she go to an emergency room if needed? Yes, if she recognized signs of serious trouble. Could we get there quickly enough? Probably.

Kim stayed at school. Resiliency, normalcy, and routine, along with appropriate flexibility, will positively influence adjustment to serious illness.

Another mother also eloquently described resiliency along a continuum. When asked how her daughter was doing after a serious motor vehicle accident that left her with back injuries and bowel and bladder problems, she said, "She's doing great but she's not finished yet." Her daughter wasn't trying to hide anything; she had accepted her physical limitations, but she was on her way to "finding a new normal."

## Death and Grief

Everyone dies. We know that. But as in the Kenny Chesney song, "everybody wants to go to heaven but nobody wants to go now." Some sobering statistics (Dean, McClement, Bond, Daeninck, & Nelson, 2005):

- Approximately one-third of adult child deaths are anticipated.
- About 10% of parents older than 60 have lost a child.
- A woman older than 65 has a 25% chance that her adult son will die before her.

This 2005 study by Dean and colleagues seems to confirm that parents of adult children who are dying are often overlooked by the healthcare professionals. Parents felt that no one could understand the loss of a child if they have not experienced it.

This study also found that helpful coping strategies during a serious illness included professional support and counseling, information about their child's illness, and faith (Dean et al., 2005). Other coping strategies included keeping memories of the dead child alive, talking about the dead child, staying connected with the grandchildren if there were any, and helping others who are having the same experience.

The ambiguities of being in an untenable situation for these parents seemed to be illustrated by their expression of disappointment that they were not acknowledged by healthcare professionals and that sometimes even well-intentioned comments by these same professionals were felt to be annoying. One father reflected that a nurse would say, "'Oh, and she's so young.' I hate that. What's that got to do with it? It's got nothing to do with it" (Dean et al., 2005, p. 759). This account perhaps reflects that no matter the age, a child's illness and death are difficult.

Any serious illness is difficult. Helping your seriously ill adult child is also difficult and often unplanned. But what if the unthinkable does happen? A question that continues to haunt Sandra Cesario is (personal communication, October 8, 2010):

> "What do you call a childless mother?" Yes, she is always a mother, but how do you distinguish her from other mothers who have living children? A wife is a widow after her husband dies; a child is an orphan after his parents die. What is a mother after her child dies? I am not sure that labels are always good but sometimes if you have a word that you can define— a word that describes or that sets you apart—that might bring you out of the shadows. This word would help acknowledge your pain and the loss. I personally think that a word would help. A lot of parents will get to the point where they do outlive their children, what are you called?

Dr. Mohammad Alnsour, a medical oncologist in Toledo, Ohio, relates a very old Arabic word, *thakla*. This would translate to mean "mother who is crying or a grieving parent." "It is a very sad word," he says, "and not used very often. It is more of poetry. I wish there were a term" (M. Alnsour, personal communication, October 18, 2010). There is no English equivalent.

A mother whose child had died many years ago tells about the social awkwardness. "It is always awkward when meeting someone new, even after all this time. When the question inevitably comes up, 'How many children do you have?' How do I answer? Do I say three, leaving Cody out, or do I say four but one died? It's always uncomfortable."

Compassionate Friends (www.compassionatefriends.org), an organization that helps families who have lost a child, recognizes another aspect of the death of an adult child: Many parents have developed a friendship with their grown child. Not only have they lost their child but also a friend, sometimes even a best friend. Compassionate Friends (n.d.) recommends the following.

- Talk about the death, the loss, and the pain. Revisit good memories of your child and not just the immediate memories of death.
- Allow friends to help. They are sincere when they ask, "What can I do?"
- Consider doing something constructive in memory of your child, some sort of a memorial. Some parents have established memorial funds, created scholarships, made donations to special charities, planted trees, and donated books. It helps to help others, parents have often advised.

There is no better or worse way to lose a child. There is no better or worse age to lose a child. In a very real sense, parents make a total commitment to raising their children. This is their life's work. It is an important lifetime investment in time, love, and energy. An old saying goes, "Our children are living messages we send to a time and place we will never see." With the death of an adult child, their life work dies.

Ann Finkbeiner interviewed parents after the death of an adult child. Her 1998 book relates stories with many parents poignantly quoted. Some of these are instructive.

- Walter, whose 18-year-old son was killed in a motor vehicle accident nine years earlier, explains two things: "Number one is that death is final. There's nothing more final in the world than death. There's no way of ever bringing him back. It's final. And the other thing is life does go on. You have to realize there are other things in life. Takes a long time to feel that way" (Finkbeiner, 1998, p. 3).
- After the death of a loved one, people experience searching behavior. The concept of searching behavior refers to searching for someone who's died. One may expect to "see" them on the street or at the mall or eating at a favorite restaurant or sitting in church, whatever might have been their habit. This is common with all close deaths, but parents seem to have extra reason for searching. They always expected to die before their children. A parent dying first is the natural order of the world; "a world in which you are alive and your child is not feels unnatural. Your child isn't here so you shouldn't be; . . . you feel 'out of place.' You're still here so the child must be too; and so . . . you search" (Finkbeiner, 1998, p. 6).
- Is suicide after the death of a child, or thoughts of suicide, a parent's way of following or going after the child who died? Early in their grief, parents didn't so much choose to live; they just didn't choose to die. Choosing to live comes later.

Research by Weed (2007) attempted to better understand the experience of parents after the death of an adult child. In an article titled "Lifelong Hurt," she describes that these parents' lives are changed forever. Even when not directly asked, each of the participants described the meaning of the experience in meticulous detail beginning with the events that led up to the death. It was as if to understand the experience, one needed to know about the child's life and events that led to the death.

Author Jeanne Webster Blank (1998) discerns that an adult child is the finished product, one that will go into the future, create a legacy. A young child is potential; the loss is one of what might have been. In a sense, with an adult child the memoir is written and the pictures are in the book—Christmases, many of them; graduations, perhaps multiple; even marriages and grandchildren. She contends that it is also this life project and these memories that can provide comfort after a death. They are comforting to have, she says from experience, but like all bereaved parents, she still would rather have her daughter back alive. In that, the age of a lost child does not matter.

Chaplain, social worker, and therapist Kathy Capps observed that at the time of death, love doesn't end but changes form. She said, "The love remains in stories and in the faces of children and grandchildren" (personal communication, October 29, 2011).

## Advance Care Planning

Serious illness does sometimes help mend relationships, observed Dr. Alnsour (personal communication, October 18, 2010). Parents are more likely to forgive their children than with other relationships. "Often it is the mothers who reach out to mend relationships; fathers are more likely to forgive their daughters than their sons," he said.

He elaborated further,

> The first thing to understand is that the patient will go through the phases of grief. They will be angry and in denial. A lot of times the patient and the parents have some form of an explosive confrontation at this time; shouting at each other, perhaps saying hurtful things. The challenge is to be supportive and understand that this is a phase. The anger will go away and may be followed by bargaining or depression. If the parents are able to get through the anger phase, patients do not start reaching out to their parents until that denial/anger phase is gone; they then start understanding. This is serious, and they might not be cured or survive. They may start to understand about legacy and leaving this life on good terms." (M. Alnsour, personal communication, October 18, 2010)

At its best, advance care planning is a conversation. This conversation takes place over time and with people who are involved with the decision making, including loved ones and healthcare professionals. Often the understanding of what is important is reached. The best of these conversations are consistent with one's values. Decisions made are consistent with how people have lived their lives. Unfortunately most people want to ignore these difficult talks because they are uncomfortable and can be sad, particularly if the outcome might be death.

Advance care planning is about respect for the human dignity of a person. It is a process that communicates those decisions and may include written advance directives. It is important because

- Most of us will die under the care of health professionals.
- Up to 50% of people cannot make their own decisions when they are near death.
- Health professionals typically treat when uncertain of the person's wishes.
- Without this discussion, loved ones have a significant chance of not knowing a person's wishes.

## Benefit Versus Burden

One way that many people make these difficult decisions is by weighing the pros and cons. It is the way many decisions are made throughout life. The ethical term for this process is called *benefit versus burden*. The individual always makes the determination of benefit versus burden. Different people may come up with different determinations for same or similar circumstances. In addition, some things are benefits under some circumstances and burdens under others. There is no one right or wrong determination.

Some would consider the following points characteristic of a benefit. Again, this is determined by the individual or surrogate. Some examples of possible benefits are

- Effective in prolonging life
- Effective in restoring or maintaining function
- Consistent with life goals and values
- Consistent with religious and cultural beliefs.

Conversely, burdens are also determined by the individual or surrogate. These possible examples may include

- Result in more or intolerable pain

- Damage body image or function
- Be psychologically harmful
- Have an unacceptable cost for the patient, including financial cost.

A most important discussion at these times very often revolves around cardiopulmonary resuscitation (CPR). A decision about CPR may or may not need to be made by a surrogate. The decision may or may not need to be made by a parent. It is never an easy decision. Here are some of the facts associated with CPR (Ramenofsky & Weissman, n.d.):

- The success rate of CPR is often thought to be much higher than it actually is. Very often television gives unrealistic expectations.
- Approximately 13%–17% of hospitalized patients survive and return to their previous level of functioning. However, success rates are much lower in some populations. For example, in the long-term care and advanced cancer populations, the success rate is well below 15%.
- Complications of CPR include prolonged hospitalization and stay in an intensive care unit on mechanical ventilation, decreased mental functioning, and fractured ribs.

## Documents

Ideally, after conversations about advance care planning and end-of-life care, decisions are documented. These decisions can also be honored if a person makes a verbal statement about his wishes or they are written in any formal or informal fashion, and some standard forms are used. Forms and laws differ by state, but the spirit of the documents is usually respected even if the forms differ. More information can be found at National Hospice and Palliative Care Organization (www.nhpco.org) or Five Wishes (www.agingwithdignity.org/five-wishes.php).

Standard advance directives documents and a brief explanation of each follow.

- *Living wills* describe individual preferences for medical treatment in cases of terminal illness or permanent incapacity. A living will is prepared while one has decisional capacity.

- A *surrogate decision maker*, also sometimes called a *durable power of attorney for health care* (often written as DPOA/HC) or *healthcare power of attorney* (often written as HC-POA), is someone appointed by the patient to make care-related decisions. Key points include the following.
  - The surrogate/proxy document can be revoked or changed at any time.
  - The surrogate only applies in the event of incapacity or inability of an individual to make his own healthcare decisions.
  - It is not financial power of attorney.
  - It is broader than a living will and not limited to terminal illness or a permanently unconscious situation.
  - Questions to ask regarding the qualifications for a surrogate: Is he willing to act as surrogate? Does he know the preferences and values of whom he represents? Will he honor or follow the plan if one has been established? Is he able to make difficult choices?

- *Physician Order for Code Status.* May also be referred to by a number of terms or acronyms: Do Not Resuscitate (DNR), Do Not Attempt Resuscitation (DNAR), No Code, and Allow Natural Death (AND). All acronyms confirm that if cardiopulmonary arrest occurs, the patient or surrogate wants no resuscitative measures to be attempted. This advance directive requires a written physician order to be legally followed by all healthcare team members, including emergency medical personnel.

- *Physician Orders for Life-Sustaining Treatment* (POLST) is another way that advance directives are being reported and respected. POLST and *Medical Orders for Life-Sustaining Treatment* (MOLST) are templates of advance care planning documents that can be tailored to reflect specific healthcare wishes for an individual after discussion or conversation. Completed in collaboration with a physician, advanced practice nurse, or physician's assistant, POLST generally documents wishes and orders regarding CPR, use of antibiotics, artificial nutrition and hydration, and other medical interventions. For more information, go to Physician Orders for Life Sustaining Treatment Paradigm (www.ohsu.edu/polst) (Meier & Beresford, 2009).

- *First-Person Consent for Organ Donation* is a specific advance directive that gives permission for organ donation. Often these are completed at the license bureau through each state's department of motor vehicles. This consent can be declared when an individual renews a driver's license.

All advance care planning decisions should be made carefully, thoughtfully, and usually with more than one conversation.

## Bonnie's Story

Through both daughters' illnesses, Bonnie has also had to watch their dreams change, and in some cases, destruct. Mary lost custody of her children; Kelly had to forfeit an invitation to officiate at a national sporting event, something she had worked to achieve for more than two decades.

Advice for others has been hard-won, but she says, "Respect for your child's decisions, including their partner, must always guide your actions." Sometimes this will mean that you change your strategy of helping, you wait to be asked, and you practice restraint.

Finally, "take care of yourself." She recalled that shortly after the accident, she received a scolding from a friend for taking a walk alone, for leaving Mary's bedside. "What did my friend know? How could she ever put herself in my place?" Rejuvenation and energy are necessary for caregivers to continue doing what is needed—providing love and support during serious illness and asking questions. Indeed, who can tell someone else how to behave in these unthinkable circumstances?

"You make the best decisions you can at the time," Bonnie says with the wisdom of someone who has been baptized into this growing and not so invisible group of parents with seriously ill adult children.

## Conclusion

Sometimes getting out of bed in the morning is hard because of the fear of how the day will affect your child. The outcomes of a serious illness are only one part of the answer to the important question, "What next?" There are many answers to this question. The people in this book each had a unique story, each was different than anyone else, different than any other family. But patterns and themes emerged. One of these is love.

In fact, among the assumptions made in this book, that you love your child looms largest. There are other types of parent-child relationships, but because you picked up this book, yours is probably a loving one. And now, through some unknown power in the universe, your adult child is seriously ill. "How did this happen?" is not a question this book answers. But, "How can I help my child?" is.

Having an ill child of any age is difficult. Before reading a page in this book, you may have discovered the power of presence. Perhaps accompanying your child is where you started. This instinct is to be honored throughout your child's illness. As Jefri Ann Franks (2010) said, "To companion the suffering is an act of courage" (p. 332). Many needs are associated with a serious illness. The approaches come down to respect. Respect for your child as an adult.

When discussing the book project with a dear friend whose daughter had been seriously ill, there was a point in the telephone conversation when she was just silent. Then she spoke, "When Sara was ill, I didn't know who to talk to . . . there was nothing out there." She and the other parents in this book asked that their stories be shared in the hope that their perspectives will help you find some guidance to support your ill adult child and yourself. They wanted you to know that you are not alone. Their stories are told to help you move out of the shadows.

> *Stories make us more alive, more human, more coura-geous, more loving. . . . Honor your own stories and tell them too. The tales may not seem very important, but they are what binds families and makes each of us who we are.*
>
> —Madeleine L'Engle

# References

Blank, J.W. (1998). *The death of an adult child: A book for and about bereaved parents.* Amityville, NY: Baywood Publishing.

Bush, N.J. (2010). Post-traumatic stress disorder related to cancer: Hope, healing, and recovery. *Oncology Nursing Forum, 37,* E331–E343. doi:10.1188/10. ONF.E331-E343

Christakis, N.A., & Lamont, E.B. (2000). Extent and determinants of error in physicians' prognoses in terminally ill patients. *Western Journal of Medicine, 172,* 310–313. Retrieved from http://www.ncbi.nlm.nih.gov/pmc/articles/PMC1070876/

Compassionate Friends. (n.d.). To the newly bereaved. Retrieved from http://www.compassionatefriends.org/Find_Support/Personal-Note/To_the_Newly_Bereaved.aspx

Dean, M., McClement, S., Bond, J.B., Jr., Daeninck, P.J., & Nelson, F. (2005). Parental experiences of adult child death from cancer. *Journal of Palliative Medicine, 8,* 751–765. doi:10.1089/jpm.2005.8.751

Edwards, E. (2009). *Resilience: Reflections on the burdens and gifts of facing life's adversities.* New York, NY: Crown Publishing Group.

Finkbeiner, A.K. (1998). *After the death of a child: Living with loss through the years.* Baltimore, MD: Johns Hopkins University Press.

Franks, J.A. (2010). The power of presence. *Journal of Palliative Medicine, 13,* 331–332. doi:10.1089/jpm.2009.0313

Katz, A. (2012). *After you ring the bell ... Ten challenges for the cancer survivor.* Pittsburgh, PA: Hygeia Media.

Meier, D.E., & Beresford, L. (2009). POLST offers next stage in honoring patient preferences. *Journal of Palliative Medicine, 12,* 291–295. doi:10.1089/jpm.2009.9648

Ramenofsky, D.H., & Weissman, D.E. (n.d.). #179 CPR survival in the hospital setting. Retrieved from http://www.eperc.mcw.edu/EPERC/FastFactsIndex/ff_179.htm

Taylor, J.B. (2008). *My stroke of insight: A brain scientist's personal journey.* New York, NY: Viking.

Weed, L.D. (2007). Lifelong hurt: Older parents' experience after the death of an adult child. *Journal of Hospice and Palliative Nursing, 9,* 22–30.

Yourman, L.C., Lee, S.J., Schonberg, M.A., Widera, E.W., & Smith, A.K. (2012). Prognostic indices for older adults: A systematic review. *JAMA, 307,* 182–192. doi:10.1001/jama.2011.1966

**By the Way...**

- Advance care planning is about discussions; the conversations we have with those we love about our wishes for end-of-life care. It extends to the documents that we complete.
- The American Society of Clinical Oncology offers *Cancer Survivorship: Next Steps for Patients and Their Families* (www.cancer.net/survivorship), which includes ideas and examples for a survivor care plan.
- Allow friends to help. They are sincere when they ask, "What can I do?"
- If there is a death, talk about the loss and the pain. Revisit good memories and not just the immediate memories of death. Consider doing something constructive in memory of your child, some sort of a memorial. Memories, pictures, and memoirs can be a comfort but they do not replace the wish for the lost child to be back alive.
- Cancer*Care* (www.cancercare.org) encourages you to treat yourself with kindness and patience, take care of your health, plan ahead for how to cope with special days, share your feelings, gather favorite photos, create a special remembrance, seek comfort in your spiritual beliefs, keep a journal, consider professional help, and consider a support group.

# Appendix

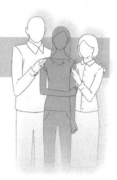

## Helping to Relieve Pain and Other Symptoms

### Aromatherapy
- Description: Aromatherapy is the controlled use of plant essences for therapeutic purposes.
- How aromatherapy helps: Essential oils are the aromatic essences of plants in the form of oil or resin that has been extracted in highly concentrated solutions. They are thought to have antiviral, antiseptic, antibacterial, anti-inflammatory, fungicidal, sedative, and anticongestive properties.
- Special considerations and precautions: Often practiced with massage, essential oils should not be administered orally or applied undiluted to the skin. Contraindications include contagious disease, venous thrombosis, open wounds, and recent surgery.
- Equipment: Essential oils
- Directions: Aromatherapy is used in various ways. Examples include the following.
  - Indirect inhalation: The person breathes in essential oils by using a room diffuser or placing drops nearby, such as on bed linens or in a container on a nightstand.
  - Direct inhalation: The person breathes in essential oils by using an individual inhaler with drops floated on top of hot water.
  - Aromatherapy massage: A caregiver or professional massage therapist can massage essential oils, diluted in a carrier oil such as grape seed, sweet almond, olive, or other nonfragrant oils, into the skin.
  - Essential oils can be applied to the skin by combining them with bath salts, lotions, or dressings.

## Massage

- Description: Massage is the stroking or rubbing of the skin surface for pain relief or relaxation.
- How massage helps: Massage can be used to decrease pain by soothing the skin and relaxing tense muscles.
- Special considerations and precautions: Do not massage areas treated with radiation because the skin is very delicate, an open skin wound or sore or one that is healing, areas too sensitive to touch, or if massage increases pain. Massage should not be used directly over an area of a tumor or over any area with bone metastasis.
- Equipment: Massage oil or powder and a large towel or blanket
- Directions: The most common areas for massage are the back and shoulders, but if this is too uncomfortable, a foot or hand rub may be just as relaxing. Choose the area that is best for the person receiving the massage.
  - Remove clothing from the area to be massaged.
  - For warmth and privacy, cover the parts of the body not being massaged.
  - Use powder or oil, whichever is preferred, just to keep the movement smooth. Friction caused by rubbing the skin without lotion can cause more irritation and discomfort. If lotion is used, warm it first by placing it in the microwave for a few seconds or by placing the bottle in a pan of warm water. Test the lotion first before placing it on the skin.
  - Choose the time carefully; before the pain becomes severe and when the person is tired or anxious are often good opportunities for massage to be helpful. Set aside a time each day for a massage.
  - The length of time for the massage depends on the individual. A few minutes may be all that is necessary to obtain results.
  - Use long, firm strokes in the area being massaged. If the hands and feet are massaged, rub each finger and toe separately.
  - Ask the person, "What feels good? Are softer strokes more relaxing? Firmer strokes?" It is important to have the person tell you what is best.
  - Massage is a time to relax. Just concentrate on how the massage feels to the person and avoid talking and other noise.
  - To help them relax, some people like to have their favorite music playing while they receive a massage.
  - Massage is not intended to take the place of pain medication; it is meant to work with the medication to help achieve better pain relief.

## Distraction: Music

* Description: Distraction is a means of using the senses (hearing, seeing, touch, and movement) to focus attention on something other than pain. One method of distraction is the use of music, if this is acceptable and enjoyable to the person.
* How music helps: When distraction is used, pain is more bearable and the person's mood is better because he or she is not concentrating on the pain. There is more control over the pain sensation.
* Equipment: There are many different ways to listen to music, including CD player, MP3 player, computer, or radio. The listener can choose to enjoy the music with headphones or use speakers to create ambiance throughout a room. Choose what is familiar, available, and comfortable to use.
* Directions
  - Decide what type of music is enjoyed.
  - Find a comfortable room and a comfortable position.
  - If possible, use distraction when the pain starts, before it becomes severe. Have the person take pain medication, and listen to the music as the medication starts to work.
  - Try to have the person either sing along with the music or tap his or her fingers and feet to the beat.
  - The more senses used—touch, hearing—the more the individual will think about what he or she is doing and may be able to take thoughts away from the pain. Again, this does not mean that the pain is not severe or real, but research has shown that distraction techniques are powerful in making even severe pain more bearable.
  - Try to use this method of distraction several times a day for best results.
  - Distraction does not take the place of pain medication; it is meant to work with the medication to help achieve better pain relief.

## Distraction: Humor

* Description: As mentioned previously, distraction is a means of using the senses to focus attention on something other than pain. Another method of distraction is the use of humor.
* How humor helps: Studies have shown that laughter helps decrease stress, promotes relaxation, boosts the immune system, releases endorphin or the body's natural "feel-good" chemicals, and improves blood flow.
* Equipment: Many different audio and video equipment are available such as a CD player, MP3 player, computer, or radio. Books, maga-

zines, or electronic reading devices such as a Nook® or Kindle® can also be used. Most smartphones and tablets also have the ability to stream audio or video material. Choose what is familiar, available, and comfortable to use.

- Directions
  - Decide what type of comedy is enjoyed the most. Is it a favorite sitcom on TV? A funny movie? A favorite book?
  - Find a comfortable room and a comfortable position.
  - If possible, use distraction when the pain starts, before it becomes severe. Suggest taking pain medication and listen or watch as the medication starts to work.
  - Try not to have any interruptions while the person is listening or watching his or her favorite comedy material.
  - The more senses used— sight, touch, hearing—the more the individual will think about what he or she is doing and may be able to take thoughts away from the pain. Again, this does not mean that the pain is not severe or real. But research has shown that distraction techniques are powerful in making even severe pain more bearable.
  - Try to use this method of distraction several times a day.
  - Distraction does not take the place of pain medication; it is meant to work with the medication to help achieve better pain relief.

**Relaxation: Guided Imagery**
- Description: Relaxation is resting to achieve a reduction in tension. One method of relaxation is the use of guided imagery. Imagery is using imagination to help lessen pain. It is a way of "picturing" a thought or image that will distract from pain.
- How guided imagery helps: Relaxation is used to help reduce stress that can cause muscle tension. Relaxation itself may not decrease pain, but rather it can help relieve tense muscles that may be contributing to the pain and help cope with all that is happening. It also functions as distraction with the benefits of focusing attention elsewhere besides on a physical symptom.
- Special considerations and precautions: Do not use deep breathing and imagery techniques if the individual has difficulty breathing or has other medical problems with the lungs.
- Equipment: A room that is comfortable and private
- Directions
  - Find a quiet room where the individual can get into a comfortable position to relax. Ask him to close his eyes.
  - Ask the person to not fold his arms or cross his legs because it may cut off circulation and cause numbness and tingling.

- Instruct the person to breathe in deeply and exhale slowly as though whistling out. The individual should do this three times. This will help him to relax.
- Have the individual picture in his mind something that is peaceful or a place that he has enjoyed visiting.
- Have him think of an image that is pleasant and symbolizes pain relief.
  * For example, if the person thinks of pain as being a large boulder that is on a part of the body weighing him down and causing pain, perhaps he can picture large helium filled balloons attached to the boulder carrying it away and releasing the pain.
  * Perhaps he may think of the pain as a thunderstorm, complete with lightning and thunder, that rains on the body. He can imagine how the pain medication is like a gentle breeze that blows the rain and thunderclouds away. Instead of rain and thunder, suggest that he visualize sunshine and warmth. The air smells clean and fresh, the rain has watered all the beautiful flowers, and the grass is green and lush. There are swans and ducks on a pond. Only a ripple, caused by the ducks' gentle paddling, disturbs the water's peaceful state.
- Use guided imagery at least 20 minutes a day. It is best if this is tried before the pain becomes severe, or while waiting for the pain medication to work.
- Imagery is not intended to take the place of pain medication; it is meant to work with the medication to help achieve better pain relief.

## Relaxation: Breathing Exercises
- Description: Relaxation is resting to achieve a reduction in tension. One method of relaxation is the use of breathing exercises.
- How breathing exercises help: Breathing exercises promote relaxation, which helps reduce stress that can cause muscle tension, which in turn can increase pain. The focus on controlled breathing promotes improved oxygenation and adds an element of distraction from a physical complaint. Relaxation itself may not decrease pain, but rather it can help relieve tense muscles that may be contributing to the pain and help an individual cope with all that is happening.
- Special considerations and precautions: Deep breathing techniques should not be used if the individual has difficulty breathing or has other medical problems with the lungs.

- Equipment: Many different audio and video equipment are available, including a CD player, MP3 player, computer, or radio. Choose what is familiar, available, and comfortable to use.
- Directions
  - Find a quiet room where the individual can get into a comfortable position to relax. Ask the person to close his eyes.
  - Similar to guided imagery, the person should not fold his arms or cross his legs because it may cut off circulation and cause numbness and tingling.
  - Ask the person to breathe in deeply and exhale slowly as though whistling out. Instruct the person to do this three times. This will help the person to relax.
  - Have the person think of a calm, peaceful setting, or perhaps a place that he has enjoyed visiting.
  - Instruct the person to picture his body as being very light, floating weightlessly, very limp, or comfortably warm. Use any mental picture that will promote relaxation, and then begin the breathing exercises.
  - Ask the person to breathe in deeply. At the same time, the person should tense muscles or any group of muscles you choose. For example, suggest that the person make a fist, clench the jaw, close eyes tightly, or draw the arms or legs up as tightly as possible.
  - Instruct the person to hold his breath and keep those muscles tense for a second or two and then relax those muscles. Next, the person should breathe out and let the body relax.
  - Now, instruct the person to start with the muscles in the lower legs, concentrating on one leg at a time and, alternately tightening and releasing, work up by muscle group to the head.
  - For a shorter relaxation exercise, you may combine muscle groups. For example, you can instruct the person to tense and relax the muscles in both legs together instead of each leg separately.
  - There are audiotapes or CDs available that will talk through a series of breathing exercises to help a person relax. If this method is chosen, try to concentrate on the speaker and what is being said.
  - Use relaxation at least 20 minutes a day. It is best to try this before the pain becomes severe, or while waiting for the pain medication to work.
  - Breathing exercises are not intended to take the place of pain medication; they are meant to work with the medication to help achieve better pain relief.

**Cold Therapy**
- Description; Pain relief may bc obtained by applying cold to the painful area. When cold is applied to the skin, the cold decreases skin sensations by numbing nerve endings. Cold may also reduce muscle spasms, reduce inflammation, and help stop the desire to scratch areas that itch.
- Special considerations and precautions: Do not apply an ice bag to skin being treated with radiation therapy, severe injury, a wound in the healing phase, or areas that have poor circulation. Do not use cold if pain increases.
- Equipment: Ice bag (Any of the following may be used for an ice bag: commercial ice bag; self-sealing small plastic bag that won't leak such as a sandwich or freezer bag, filled with ice; a bag of frozen corn kernels or peas); a towel or pillowcase; menthol-containing products such as Bengay® or Icy Hot®
- Directions
  - Fill the ice bag with ice. The smaller the cubes, the better. Crushcd or shavcd ice will mold around the area better than large cubes. Push out all the air from the bag. If you are using a small plastic bag rather than a commercial ice bag, be sure it does not leak by testing it first by adding water to check for holes.
  - If you are using bags of frozen vegetables, hit the bag on the countertop once or twice to break up the frozen vegetables so the bag will mold to the skin better. Place the plastic bag directly on the skin.
  - Some commercial ice bags are prefilled with chemicals that are cold when activated. Follow the directions that come with the bag and discard it when it shows signs of wear to avoid getting these chemicals on the skin.
  - Wrap the ice bag in a pillowcase or a towel. If you want it colder, use a wet towel, if you want it less cold, use a dry towel.
  - Be sure the ice bag top is screwed on tightly and that there are no leaks. Hold the bag upside down to be sure the top is on tight.
  - Place the ice bag on the area that is painful. If it is too painful to put the ice bag directly on the area, the ice bag may be placed above or below the painful area, or on the other side of the body that corresponds to where the pain is located. For example, if the right hip hurts but it is too painful to place the ice bag there, the ice bag can be placed on the left hip.
  - Move the individual to a comfortable position.

- Leave the ice bag on 10–15 minutes, three or four times a day. The longer it is left in place (up to one hour), the longer the pain relief.
- You may alternate cold with heat. You may have to try heat and cold several times to find the correct area or temperature that gives the most relief.
- Products containing menthol such as Bengay or Icy Hot can be applied to the painful area when using cold, but not with heat, as burns may occur. Wash hands thoroughly after using any product that contains menthol and avoid getting it into eyes. Try a small amount of the menthol product on the person's inner arm. If, after a few minutes, you do not see any redness or irritation, the product may be used.
- You may refreeze the bag of vegetables to use again. (Do not cook the vegetables if they have been used as an ice pack.)
- Ice bags are not intended to take the place of medication; they are meant to work with the medication to help achieve better pain relief.

**Heat Therapy: Heating Pad, Hot Water Bottle, and Hot Bath**
- Description: Heat is the application of warmth to the skin for the relief of pain. Heat can relieve pain by improving circulation to the muscles, which decreases spasms and reduces inflammation and soreness. Heat also decreases sensitivity to pain, relieves joint stiffness, and increases blood flow to the skin. Heat also helps people to relax.
- Special considerations and precautions: Heat can burn if used improperly. Use heat with caution when sensation in an area is decreased or there is any other irritation to the skin surface. Read the manufacturer's directions before using any heating pad or hot water bottle. Follow all precautions listed with heating pads to avoid electrical shock. Do not apply heat to skin being treated with radiation therapy; any area that is bleeding; any area with decreased sensation; or any injury within the first 24 hours. Do not use heating pads or hot water bottles with any menthol-containing products (Vicks®, Bengay, Icy Hot, etc.). Do not use if oxygen is being used.
- Equipment
  - Heating pad, manufacturer's cover for the heating pad
  - Hot water bottle, towel, thermometer used for swimming pools or spas, towel or pillowcase
  - Bath tub, thermometer used for swimming pools and spas, and towels

- Heating pad directions
  - Plug in the heating pad and place the temperature control on low, Adjust to a higher heat if needed.
  - When the heating pad is warm, place the heating pad on the area where the person wants relief.
  - If the area is too painful to have the heating pad directly on it, place it on the other side of the body that corresponds to the painful area. For example, if the right hip has pain but it is too painful to put the heating pad on the right hip, put the heating pad on the left hip.
  - Be certain the heating pad has a cover over it to prevent burning the skin.
  - Do not allow the person to fall asleep on top of the heating pad. Heat is increased with pressure, which may cause burns.
  - Keep the heating pad on for as long as possible to obtain relief, usually 20–30 minutes but not longer than 30 minutes.
  - Alternate heat and cold (please see the instructional materials on cold) to improve comfort. Try either heat or cold several times to find the correct area or temperature that gives the most relief.
  - If the heating pad is too warm, decrease the temperature to a lower temperature. Adjust the temperature of the heating pad for comfort. Heating pads can burn fragile skin; hotter is not always better.
  - Use the heating pad as often as necessary for relief. Try to use the heating pad before the pain becomes severe.
  - The heating pad does not take the place of pain medication; it is meant to work with the medication to help achieve better pain relief.
- Hot water bottle directions
  - Fill the hot water bottle with hot water from the faucet. Do not put boiling water into the hot water bottle.
  - Use the thermometer made for swimming pools and spas to take the temperature of the water as it runs from the tap into the hot water bottle.
  - Water temperature should be between 104°F and 113°F (40°C and 45°C).
  - Push all the air out of the hot water bottle and screw cap on tightly. Check to see that it's sealed by holding the bottle upside down.
  - Place the hot water bottle in a towel or pillowcase.
  - Place the hot water bottle on the area where relief is wanted. If it is too painful to place the hot water bottle directly on the painful area, place it above or below the painful site. It also can be placed

on the other side of the body that corresponds to the painful area. For example, if the right hip has pain but it is too painful to put the hot water bottle on the right hip, put it on the left hip.
- Do not allow the person to sleep on top of the hot water bottle. Heat is increased with pressure, which may cause burns to the skin.
- Keep the hot water bottle on for as long as possible to obtain relief, usually between 20–30 minutes. Refill with hot water when the bottle is no longer warm. Recheck temperature.
- Alternate use of the hot water bottle and switch to cold (please see the instructional materials on cold) to improve comfort. Try heat and cold several times to find the correct area or temperature that gives the person the most relief.
- Hot water bottles are not intended to take the place of pain medication; they are meant to work with the medication to help achieve better pain relief.
• Hot bath directions
- Fill the bathtub with enough warm water to cover the painful area.
- Before getting into the tub, take the temperature of the water with the thermometer.
- The water temperature should be between 98°F and 102°F (36.7°C and 38.9°C).
- The person should sit in the hot bath for as long as comfortable.
- Add more hot water as the water in the tub cools. When adding hot water, be sure to check the temperature of the water.
- Repeat tub baths as often as needed for relief. Try to initiate tub baths before the pain becomes severe.
- If pain becomes worse, if shivering occurs, or the skin becomes irritated, discontinue use of tub baths.
- Hot baths do not take the place of pain medication; they are meant to work with the medication to help achieve better pain relief.

**Tea**
• Description: Consider teas as support, comfort, and healing. No strong evidence supports that teas prevent or cure cancer. Teas are rich in antioxidants, which are absorbed to help healing and calm painful sensations. Teas are soothing if ingested or applied topically. Green teas have a reputation for being healing, white teas for calming, and both are soothing; chamomile is often used for its comforting effects. Warm compresses using teas have been used to draw out an infection and relieve pain.
• Equipment: Pot for boiling water, loose leaf tea or tea bag, infuser or strainer for loose leaf tea

- Directions for topical use
  - Prepare the tea with boiling water using the strainer for loose leaf tea.
  - Soak either towels or gauze in the tea while it cools to room temperature.
  - Apply to the skin. Do not apply to open wounds.

*Note.* Based on information from City of Hope & American Association of Colleges of Nursing. (2008). *End-of-Life Nursing Education Consortium (ELNEC) SuperCore curriculum: Module 3, Symptom management.* Washington, DC: Authors; Jackson-Michel, S. (2011, March 9). Home remedy to draw out infection. Retrieved from http://www.livestrong.com/article/218580-home-remedy-to-draw-out-infection; National Comprehensive Cancer Network. (2011). *NCCN Clinical Practice Guidelines in Oncology: Cancer-related fatigue* [v.1.2012]. Retrieved from http://www.nccn.org/professionals/physician_gls/pdf/fatigue.pdf